MW01002896

THE ART OF
NARRATIVE PSYCHIATRY

*The Art of Narrative Psychiatry* is graceful and eminently practical. Hamkins reveals through clinical tales how she has translated narrative therapy from its sources in Family Therapy, Counseling, and Social Work in to mainstream psychiatry. Her gracious practice inheres in these stories and comes alive both in the reading of them and her commentaries. This book returns to the historical concerns of psychiatry in regard to the human soul and as such provides a professional niche for those who wish to engage in such concerns rather than merely prescribe.

—David Epston, co-director, the Family Therapy Centre, Auckland, New Zealand
and co-author of *Narrative Means to Therapeutic Ends* and
*Biting the Hand that Starves You: Inspiring Resistance to Anorexia/Bulimia*

Dr. Hamkins is a wise and empathic clinician who deeply understands how the stories people tell about themselves not only describe their lives—but also shape them. *The Art of Narrative Psychiatry* is an elegantly written and vital new book, which weaves insightful clinical examples with practical guidance, and ultimately shows how understanding the power of stories can lead to an energizing and creative collaboration with patients.

—Bradley Lewis, MD, PhD, Gallatin School of Individualized Study,
New York University, NY and author of
*Narrative Psychiatry: How Stories Can Shape Clinical Practice*

Dr. SuEllen Hamkins offers a fresh alternative to psychiatrists who wish to re-invigorate their commitment to alleviating suffering in their patients. By applying principles and practices of narrative therapy to psychiatry, Dr. Hamkins describes—and then beautifully illustrates—how psychiatrists can carefully attend to the critical problems facing their patients, while simultaneously engaging with their stories of sustenance, intentionality and meaning-making. I urge you to read this groundbreaking book if you believe in psychotropic medication as a compelling option, yet yearn to move beyond a hyper-focus on neurochemistry and diagnostic categorization.

—*Peggy Sax, PhD Founder,*
http://www.reauthoringteaching.com, Middlebury, VT

With this highly anticipated book SuEllen Hamkins provides a compelling account of narrative psychiatry. In drawing on the work of White and Epston's *Narrative Therapy* and bringing in the role of human biology, she builds a bridge between everyday psychiatry and post-modern practices. This hopeful work provides an antidote to the current hyper focus on neurochemistry and diagnostic categories. I highly recommend this book which rigorously details the skills of therapeutic work based on compassionate connection and engagement with life enriching stories of strength, capacity, and meaning in the face of severe psychiatric challenges.

—Shona Russell, Co-Director,
Narrative Practices Adelaide, South Australia

# THE ART OF NARRATIVE PSYCHIATRY

SuEllen Hamkins, MD

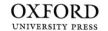

OXFORD
UNIVERSITY PRESS

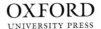

# OXFORD
## UNIVERSITY PRESS

Oxford University press is a department of the University of Oxford.
It furthers the University's objective of excellence in research, scholarship,
and education by publishing worldwide.

Oxford    New York
Auckland   Cape Town   Dar es Salaam   Hong Kong   Karachi
Kuala Lumpur   Madrid   Melbourne   Mexico City   Nairobi
New Delhi   Shanghai   Taipei   Toronto

With offices in
Argentina   Austria   Brazil   Chile   Czech Republic   France   Greece
Guatemala   Hungary   Italy   Japan   Poland   Portugal   Singapore
South Korea   Switzerland   Thailand   Turkey   Ukraine   Vietnam

Oxford is a registered trademark of Oxford University Press
in the UK and certain other countries.

Published in the United States of America by
Oxford University Press
198 Madison Avenue, New York, NY 10016

Library of Congress Cataloging-in-Publication Data
Hamkins, SuEllen, author.
The art of narrative psychiatry / by SuEllen Hamkins.
p. ; cm.
Includes bibliographical references and index.
ISBN 978–0–19–998204–2 (alk. paper) — ISBN 978–0–19–998205–9 (alk. paper) —
ISBN 978–0–19–998206–6 (alk. paper)    I.  Title.
[DNLM: 1.  Narrative Therapy—methods. WM 420]
RC489.S74
616.89'165—dc23
2013008144

The science of medicine is a rapidly changing field. As new research and clinical experience broaden
our knowledge, changes in treatment and drug therapy occur. The author and publisher of this
work have checked with sources believed to be reliable in their efforts to provide information that is
accurate and complete, and in accordance with the standards accepted at the time of publication.
However, in light of the possibility of human error or changes in the practice of medicine, neither the
author, nor the publisher, nor any other party who has been involved in the preparation or publication
of this work warrants that the information contained herein is in every respect accurate or complete.
Readers are encouraged to confirm the information contained herein with other reliable sources, and
are strongly advised to check the product information sheet provided by the pharmaceutical company
for each drug they plan to administer.

1  3  5  7  9  8  6  4  2
Printed in the United States of America
on acid-free paper

*To my beloved family, Jay, Tiama and Frani*

# CONTENTS

# ACKNOWLEDGMENTS

In bringing this book to life, I have been sustained by a community of supporters whose encouragement has made writing a joy. Thanks first to my editor, Craig Panner, for his faith in me, to James Fraleigh for graceful and meticulous copyediting, and to everyone at Oxford University Press who helped this book come into being.

The expertise, enthusiasm, and warmth of Jenifer McKenna, Jeff Fishman, Gerry Weiss, and Beth Prullage inspires and sustains me in my work and in writing about it. Josh Relin helps me stay true to what I value most about narrative practice, and his thoughtful comments improved every chapter. Meryl Cohn and Mary Beth Caschetta helped strike the spark that fired my faith in this project, and Meryl's insightful and encouraging comments on multiple drafts have been a gift. Kim Gaitskill and Nathan Somers's generous reading and incisive comments helped mold this book to speak more cogently to the needs of psychiatrists. I cherish Peggy Sax's encouragement to "join in the conversation" of creating narrative practices and her thoughtful reflections on early chapters. Barbara Montero and Pat Stacey's input on early drafts helped me bring the story of my work more vividly to life. Thanks to Alan Lorenz and Michael Clancy for help in understanding academic publishing. To Mary Beth Brooker, Susan Harris, and Karen Randall, I offer heartfelt gratitude for co-creating a warm, playful writing space. Thanks to Cindy Parrish and Karen Bivona for their unceasing inspiration, care, and faith in me; to Amy Bowes, Janice Waldron-Hansen, Erin Berard, and Stephen Spitzer for loving encouragement; to Gaylinn Greenwood for our early collaborations in interrogating hegemonic medical discourses; and to Mary Leonard for unstinting support and love.

I am indebted to Michael White and David Epston for developing rigorous, beautiful, ethical, and playful narrative practices and for all the training and encouragement they offered me over the years. David, I am so glad to have you as an ongoing guiding light; Michael, you are deeply missed. I am grateful to have studied intensively with Sallyann Roth and for her continued encouragement to apply narrative approaches to psychiatry. My training and conversations with Shona Russell, Bill Madsen, Gaye Stockell, Jill Freedman, Gene Combs, and Monica McGoldrick have inspired, challenged, and guided me. I am grateful to Ronald Diamond and Donald Spence for my first training as a psychiatrist, to Shoshana Sokoloff for our early narrative psychiatry collaborations, and to Bradley Lewis for inspiration and encouragement. Thanks to Jeffrey Geller, Andrea Stone, Carrie Sacco, Ken Talan, Ira Addes, Kim Gaitskill, Amy Champoux, and Farnsworth Lobenstine for their collegial counsel and support.

I am grateful for the support and encouragement of Harry Rockland-Miller and the staff of The Center for Counseling and Psychological Health at UMass-Amherst in the writing of this book, and for how their clinical acumen, dedication, and humor make it a pleasure to come to work. Thanks to David Browne, Jen LeFort, Donna Kellogg, Eliza McArdle, Robyn Miller, and Harry Rockland-Miller for collaborating in developing strengths-based medical records, and to Saleha Chaudhry, Chelsea Dann, Yu Dong, Laura Mackie, Julia Moss, Josh Relin, Linda Scott, and Chris Shanky for spearheading our narrative clinical consultation team.

I am indebted to each of the patients who appears in these pages for their generosity in sharing their stories.

Great thanks to David Denborough, Cheryl White, and Dulwich Centre Publications for their support. A modified portion of chapter 3 was published as "Introducing Narrative Psychiatry: Narrative Approaches to Initial Psychiatric Consultations," in *The International Journal of Narrative Therapy and Community Work* 1 (2005): 5–17. Copyright © SuEllen Hamkins. Reprinted with permission of Dulwich Centre Publications, www.dulwichcentre.com.au. A modified portion of chapter 6 was published as

"Bringing Narrative Practices to Psychopharmacology," in *The International Journal of Narrative Therapy and Community Work*, 1 (2010): 56–71. Copyright © SuEllen Hamkins. Reprinted with permission of Dulwich Centre Publications.

Most of all, I am grateful to my family: to my husband and colleague, Jay Indik, for his unfailing support in this as in all things, and for the clinical expertise and insight he brought to every draft and every page; to my children, Tiama and Frani Hamkins-Indik, for their interest, encouragement, creative metaphors, and dancing in the kitchen; and to my parents and siblings for their faith and love.

Patients who consult with psychiatrists and psychotherapists are often mired in stories of despair and failure. Maeli Taylor, whom I met as a staff psychiatrist at a community mental health center where I worked for fifteen years, was such a one. A heavyset woman of twenty-six, she sat in the wide armchair in my sparsely furnished office with her toes just touching the floor. Her round, pale face was blank, and she answered my initial questions with single words. I knew that she had recently been released from the hospital after making a suicide attempt—approximately her twentieth. She was on four psychotropic medicines, and had been in individual psychotherapy and a coping-skills group prior to and during her hospitalization. She had tried just about every psychotropic medication known. Her previous psychiatrist had left the agency, and now I was responsible for her psychiatric care. "I feel suicidal every day," she said.

I felt a sinking feeling in the pit of my stomach. I was afraid for both of us. Clearly psychotropic medicine and the scientifically proven dialectical behavior therapy[1] offered by the skilled clinicians at our clinic were not enough to help her recover. She would likely try to kill herself again, and she might succeed. In that moment twelve years ago, I was grateful that I had the inspiration of narrative therapy to guide me, which I had been studying intensively for the previous year[2] and was applying to my work as a psychiatrist. I was hopeful that this nascent "narrative psychiatry" might offer us a way forward, since the usual approaches of psychiatry were not working.

Narrative psychiatry, like narrative therapy, is animated by the idea that we experience our lives and our identities through the stories we tell about ourselves and the world. It combines the understandings that meaning is socially created, that we can question the narratives that influence us, that we are embodied creatures fortified by and beholden to our biology, and that when these ideas are gracefully combined in compassionate practice, tremendous healing is possible.

Narrative psychiatry is important to me personally because it is based on values that I cherish. First, it is deeply respectful of each person and his or her individual values, hopes, and dreams. Second, it values working collaboratively with patients as partners in treatment. Third, it is interested in questioning cultural narratives and operations of power in society that may be harmful to people. Fourth, narrative psychiatry does not let a problem obscure who the person is without the problem. It holds the view that problems and mental health symptoms are undeserved and that people are doing their best to resist them; that we all have problems and, at the same time, we have cherished morals, meaningful intentions, robust characters, magnificent talents, and vibrant souls; and that attending to those aspects of a person's experience and identity inspires growth and helps people overcome their problems and move their lives in the directions that they prefer. And fifth, narrative psychiatry never gives up hope that healing is possible.

I held these values before I began working narratively, but I could only operationalize them so far. In my work in the early 1990s as a psychiatrist at a college counseling service and at a community mental health center, I was able to see the vibrant souls and strong characters of my patients as they dealt with mental health challenges, but I was less successful in helping *them* see these things. (For example, prior to working narratively, I would have focused my treatment of Maeli Taylor on discovering the roots of her depression and trying different psychotropic medications, as I had been taught, even though these approaches had already been tried without success. I would not have known then how to effectively help Maeli honor what she found meaningful, tell the story of her strengths and hopes, and use that story to inspire additional steps to resist the depression.) Even though I had supplemented my traditional training as a psychiatrist in psychoanalytic psychotherapy and psycho-pharmacology with intensive study of family therapy, I felt I just didn't have the tools I needed to put my values into practice and be effective in the ways I wanted to be. I felt discouraged.

Then, in 1998, at a workshop offered by Michael White, I discovered narrative therapy.[3] This was just what I was looking for! Brilliant theory and a thousand tools with which to put it into practice! From its inception, narrative therapy sought ways to be helpful those with serious mental health challenges.[4] I immediately began adapting narrative therapy to my work in psychiatry.

So when Maeli Taylor said, "I feel suicidal every day," my hope was to discover the smallest signs of movement toward well-being and develop them into stories of strength and meaning that could inspire and sustain her. I asked her, "What percent of you wants to die, would you say?"

"Ninety percent."

"Okay," I said, initially disconcerted. Ninety percent was higher than I had anticipated—but at least it wasn't 100 percent, I thought, and that was where we might start. "Let's first talk about the 10 percent of you that wants to live. Is that okay?" She nodded, making eye contact with me. "Would you say that that's an improvement from when you were at your lowest?"

Maeli raised her eyebrows a quarter of an inch. She seemed surprised but intrigued by this line of questioning. "Yes."

Already we had discovered a positive development. On its own, the fact of her small improvement would offer her little traction in resisting the dominance of the depression in her life, but linked with other positive developments in a story that honored what she found meaningful, it would make a more compelling alternative. She and I went on to speak about what she valued and when she felt best. Slowly, Maeli told me about the good things in her life that she was enjoying, and then we spoke about what was difficult. The beginning of the "Recent History" section of my initial psychiatric consultation note captures the sense of our conversation that day:

Currently, Ms. Taylor reports that she has been able to reclaim more of her life from depression than she has ever been able to before. Currently, she reports that she is feeling OK and free of depression about 10% of the time and feels the presence of depression about 90% of the time. She notes she tends to feel more up when she is around her family, that is, her parents and her two younger sisters, because they are caring of her. She also tends to feel more OK when she goes to church, and she is helped both by the connection with the people there and her sense of spiritual connection. Furthermore, she notes sometimes at community college, she also feels OK, and sometimes feels OK in other contexts as well.

When the depression is more prevalent in her life, she experiences low energy, negative thoughts, increased sleep, difficulty getting out of bed, and increased eating. In addition, she experiences suicidal thoughts. At times, she has just thoughts; other times she develops actual plans, but [since her release from the hospital] she has been able to successfully resist acting on her suicidal impulses. One recent example is when she had an urge to take her life, she was able to think about the fact that she wanted to finish school and this prevented her from acting on it. She notes she is in her third semester studying to be a computer technician.

At the start of our session, Maeli's affect was predominantly depressed, but as our meeting proceeded she had moments of smiling and even laughing as we traced the history of her success in overcoming a tenacious depression and in pursuing her hopes for her life. Telling the story of her success in resisting depression in my consultation note stands in sharp contrast to the usual focus and tone of the medical record created to document an initial consultation, which typically focuses on the patient's problem and says little about successes in overcoming it.

I worked with Maeli for twelve years, applying the principles of narrative psychiatry that I will expound upon in detail in this book. Along with my treatment, she also engaged in dialectical behavioral therapy and art therapy, lived in a therapeutic residence, and had occasional hospitalizations. Maeli made gradual progress, with significant ups and downs along the way, ultimately reporting lower percentages of depression and higher percentages of feeling "okay." She eventually stopped making suicide attempts, and instead told us when she felt the suicidal urges were becoming unmanageable, so that we could help her utilize additional supports proactively. Notably, the attitude of the crisis intervention staff changed dramatically over the years in which I worked with her, moving from a hostile stance of blaming Maeli for the severity of her symptoms, to noticing and celebrating with her every small improvement in her ability to reach out for help rather than harming herself.

Together, Maeli and I highlighted moments of living well despite a terrible depression and linked those moments into a story of recovery. Here is what she wrote as a reflection after reading this introduction:

> I was very scared walking into Dr. Hamkins office for the first time. This was a new psychiatrist and I knew I would have to tell my story all over again. I was not looking forward to this. So I was very reticent and shy. I did not have to tell my story all over again though. Dr. Hamkins took a different approach. As it turned out, Dr. Hamkins concentrated more on what made me feel positive rather than what made me feel negative. Do not get me wrong, we did talk about the negative thoughts and feelings, however she concentrated on the positive ones. In our work together I recognized when I was suicidal and was able to tell the crisis team. Whether it was a phone conversation, respite, or hospitalization, I was able to get the help I needed.
>
> We made a "postcard" that I put on my fridge saying what I wanted in a life worth living: "Tolerating boredom, loneliness, and frustration is evidence of my courage, vision, and gutsy perseverance in doing something extraordinarily difficult in the service of my vision for my life: hubby and kids, lots of animals, be happy."
>
> I still have this on my fridge today.

Not only did this approach seem to make an enormous difference to Maeli, it made an enormous difference to me. Rather than being suffused with despair myself at the Herculean task of achieving remission of a seemingly intractable, life-threatening depression, in focusing on stories of success, no matter how small, my own spirit was sustained as well.

## THE BENEFITS OF NARRATIVE PSYCHIATRY

In bringing forward collaborative practices and narrative insights, narrative psychiatry infuses the theory and practice of psychiatry with a rigorous, refreshing corrective that balances the last decades' hyperfocus on neurochemistry and diagnostic categorization[5] with attention to the fullness of our patients' humanity, creativity, and intentionality. The both/and approach of narrative psychiatry means that we honor the sparkling, gritty complexity of our patients' unique stories while also judiciously offering them psychiatric resources, such as medication. Narrative psychiatry unpacks the ways in which psychopharmacologic discourses have tilted psychiatry toward mechanistic neurochemical explanations of the human spirit, while simultaneously listening closely to patients' experiences of the ways in which medicine has—or has not—helped them. The truth is, despite current controversies in the field, all along we in practice have been trying to be good, caring doctors and therapists who attend to our patients' humanity and want to help alleviate their suffering. Narrative psychiatry offers us new tools for doing so.

In working with patients who find psychotropic medicines to be a useful resource for alleviating symptoms and suffering, we can collaborate in finding the medicines that are the most helpful and least problematic. That said, narrative psychiatry reminds us that medicine is not the basis of someone's ability to take successful action. Such success is due to the person's talents, abilities, values, and vision. The medicine may be making those abilities and intentions more available to the person, but it does not impart the vision to pursue higher education, the ability to wire a circuit board, or the commitment to pursue spiritual development. As we pull out our prescription pads or log on to send electronic orders to a pharmacy, we can dissuade our patients from ascribing their successes to medicine and instead invite them to notice how their intentions and abilities are making the achievement of their goals possible.

In addition to its usefulness when working with patients such as Maeli who are facing the most severe psychiatric challenges, narrative psychiatry offers perspectives and tools that are useful across the range of treatment settings in which psychiatrists and psychotherapists are practicing today. Its nuanced attention to seeking stories of strength and meaning opens up new avenues for healing in our work of doing psychotherapy, whether in private practice or elsewhere. For the many contexts in which we don't have the resource of a weekly fifty-minute hour, narrative psychiatry shows us how we can bring a more healing therapeutic stance to our work, such as when our role is the busy attending doctor or social worker for an inpatient unit or at a community mental health center. Rather than focusing on a rarified look at narrative approaches in an idealized context, I am committed to developing narrative psychiatry for all the treatment contexts of psychiatry, including those that are available to patients with limited resources—that is, to most of the people who consult with psychiatrists and psychotherapists. As you will see in the chapters to come, narrative psychiatry has the power to help a lot happen in a short amount of time. In addition, it can blend with and enrich our existing ways of working. Whether we are dealing with the productivity demands of a community mental health center, the session limits of our patients' HMOs, or the spaciousness of weekly open-ended psychotherapy, narrative psychiatry offers us ways to bring greater healing to our work—and to have more satisfaction doing it.

I have found dramatic benefits from working narratively. First, the people who consult with me have steadier and more rapid success in overcoming their problems. Second, I and the people who consult with me enjoy collaborative and mutually respectful relationships. Third, it's way more fun! Instead of feeling weighed down by my patients' problems, I feel buoyed and inspired by their successes in overcoming them.

Empirical evidence for the efficacy of narrative approaches to mental health treatment is accruing. In addition to a wealth of case-based and qualitative research,[6] quantitative evidence-based studies have been completed[7] and more are currently underway.[8] Notably, narrative research seeks to collaborate with patients in assessing treatment efficacy. In addition, "co-research" by patients and doctors about the nature of the problems patients are facing and what is and isn't helping to relieve their suffering is part of every treatment.[9] My hope is that this book will inspire additional studies.

## THE ORIGINS AND CONTEXT OF NARRATIVE PSYCHIATRY

Personally, I can trace the origins of narrative psychiatry as I theorize and practice it as arising from the confluence of several streams of inspiration in my life. In college, my studies in postmodern philosophy[10] and feminist theory[11] gave me the tools of narrative analysis and inspired me early on to discern and unpack operations of power in society. I studied medicine with the intention of becoming a doctor who could selectively draw from biomedical discourses while resisting their hegemony, with hopes of attending more empathically to my patients. I studied psychiatry with the hope of finding ways to bring healing to the human soul, while resisting psychiatry's reductionistic and paternalistic tendencies. Narrative psychotherapy[12] gave me a playground of ideas, a workshop full of therapeutic tools, and a community of colleagues, including other psychiatrists interested in narrative approaches.

Concurrent with my development as a narrative psychiatrist, other psychiatrists were also inspired by narrative theory and by humanistic and collaborative values, and developed ideas for how to approach the practice of psychiatry from a narrative perspective. Gene Combs helped develop narrative therapy from its inception as exemplified in the book he coauthored with Jill Freedman, *Narrative Therapy: The Social Construction of Preferred Realities* (1996),[13] and he uses narrative approaches in his practice of psychiatry,[14] although he does not emphasize narrative psychiatry in his writings or presentations. I began developing narrative psychiatry in 1998, and published two articles about my work in *The International*

*Journal of Narrative Therapy and Community Work:* "Introducing Narrative Psychiatry: Narrative Approaches to Initial Psychiatric Consultations" in 2005, and "Bringing Narrative Approaches to Psychopharmacology" in 2010.[15] Lewis Mehl-Madrona, in *Healing the Mind through the Power of Story: The Promise of Narrative Psychiatry* (2010),[16] discusses narrative theory as it applies to psychiatry and tells how he brings the power of compassion, collaboration, cultural awareness, and personal and indigenous storytelling to his practice of psychiatry in rural Canada. Bradley Lewis, in *Narrative Psychiatry: How Stories Can Shape Clinical Practice* (2011),[17] describes the ways that narrative medicine, narrative therapy, and the narrative integration of different types of psychotherapy pave the way for a narratively attuned psychiatric practice.

So how shall we tell the story of where narrative psychiatry comes from? Here is a short version that I find useful. In a nutshell,[18] contemporary recognition of the importance of narrative in constructing our experiences arose first in philosophy, exemplified by the work of the so-called postmodern French philosophers Michel Foucault[19] and Paul Ricoeur,[20] who demonstrated the power of narrative to constrain or liberate human perceptions, understandings, and hopes. *Postmodern* refers to the recognition that while it is grounded in reality, all of human knowledge—what we consider to be "true," including science and medicine—is influenced by the narrative perspectives and social privileges of its creators.[21] Postmodern narrative theory then infused other branches of the humanities, leading to a narrative turn in the arts, literature, anthropology, and theatre,[22] ultimately permeating the clinical realm of psychotherapy, as exemplified in the work of Michael White and David Epston. The originators of what came to be known as narrative therapy, their ideas became widely disseminated following the publication of their book *Narrative Means to Therapeutic Ends* in 1990.[23] Simultaneously, human rights and social justice movements, such as feminism,[24] used the tools of postmodern narrative theory, such as analyzing social discourses to see whom they benefit, to deconstruct oppressive operations of power. Concomitantly, narrative literary theory, in combination with humanistic approaches to medicine, inspired narrative medicine, as popularized by Rita Charon's work and her lyrical book *Narrative Medicine: Honoring Stories of Illness,* published in 2006.[25] Psychiatrists such as Mehl-Madrona, Combs, and I began applying the approaches of narrative therapy in our psychiatric work.[26] Given this historical and clinical context, narrative psychiatry can be seen as the child of narrative therapy and psychiatry, the sibling of narrative medicine, and the grandchild of postmodern philosophy, narrative theory, humanistic medicine, and social justice movements.

But of course psychiatry has always attended carefully to the narratives that patients tell about their lives. In this, it is similar to narrative medicine,[27] which honors patients' stories and not just their symptoms. What distinguishes narrative psychiatry from both psychiatry-as-usual and narrative medicine is that it focuses in particular on discovering and fleshing out stories of *strength and meaning*—stories that are implicit in the patient's presenting narrative, but that may have been unrecognized and, as yet, untold[28]. (It was just this kind of untold story that I had hoped to elicit in my conversations with Maeli Taylor.)

Narrative psychiatry deepens the insights of postmodern narrative theory that inform the field of narrative medicine. Narrative psychiatry understands that the stories of illness or suffering that our patients bring to us arise in relational contexts influenced by cultural discourses that may or may not promote our patients' well-being, and that there are many stories that might be told about what they are experiencing. Therefore, in addition to attending to and being moved by the narratives that patients first tell, narrative psychiatry seeks to discover and flesh out new narratives implicit in their experiences that honor their strengths and values while also exposing and disqualifying the narratives that are damaging. Furthermore, narrative psychiatry takes particular care to honor the patient's values, preferences, and perspectives—putting the patient in the position of being the expert on his or her life—and to resist imposing the values and perspectives of the doctor. Honoring patients' personal values and strengths while remaining emotionally attuned to their suffering and joy allows the psychiatrist to offer patients a deeply felt sense of empathy and compassion.

Narrative psychiatry is distinct from narrative therapy in that it explicitly includes the role of human biology in its theory. Although the stories we tell about our bodies' biological talents and misfortunes greatly influence our experiences, our bodies have a physical existence that is not mediated by story or narrative. Learning to ride a bike, drinking a glass of wine, breaking a leg, having a stroke, and metabolizing neurotransmitters are examples of physical aspects of living in a body. Narrative psychiatry shares with narrative medicine the explicit appreciation of the importance of biology in influencing our experiences. At the same time, narrative psychiatry values investigating and questioning the narratives about biology that are influencing us.

Narrative psychiatry, like narrative therapy, differs from typical psychoanalytic and much of cognitive-behavioral psychotherapy in that it focuses on seeking the sources of a person's strength, rather than on finding the root of their problems. While narrative psychiatry stays attuned to patients' experiences of their problems, it emphasizes conversations that provide answers to questions such as, *What is helping you get through this difficult time?* and *What are the roots of that strength or value in your childhood?* rather than conversations that seek answers to questions such as, *Why are you having this problem?* or *What are the roots of this problem in your childhood?*

## THIS BOOK

I have written this book to bring narrative psychiatry to life. It is a practical book about practice and it is a theoretically rigorous book that relishes ideas. It slows down to look at what therapeutically unfolds moment by moment between a patient and a psychiatrist as they cocreate new narratives that open up fresh possibilities for well-being. In every chapter, you will see narrative psychiatry in action and you will be offered tools you can immediately put to use.

A word about the word *patient*. I find that its origins as one who *suffers, endures,* and *perseveres*[29] honors the experience of those who consult with us and emphasizes that our responsibility to them is larger than that of financial interest, as words like *clients* or *consumers* imply.

I am grateful that so many of my patients have given me permission to share the stories of our work together in this book. In many cases, my patient has read the chapter in which he or she appears and has been invited to offer corrections and reflections, several of which are included. The one exception to my practice of obtaining explicit permission to write about my patients is the story of the elderly Mrs. Eason, with whom I worked as an intern over two decades ago and who moved me to write about her in my journal at the time. She appears in chapter 2; I changed any identifying features. I use pseudonyms for everyone (most patients chose their own pseudonym) and I have changed identifying details to protect privacy.

This book is intended as an introduction, and while it addresses core narrative concepts, it is not exhaustive. In part I, the first chapter offers an overview, then chapters 2 through 6 each focus on a core element of narrative psychiatry, offering the reader a foundation for narrative practice. In part II, chapters 7 through 9 bring together the elements of narrative psychiatry, looking with more depth and nuance at narrative practice in the context of a complex case. Further exploration of these ideas and practices is needed to fully flesh out what narrative psychiatry is and can be.

This book is about healing. Narrative psychiatry is a deeply respectful, creative, and effective way to practice psychiatry, a way that empathically attends to the power of story in our lives. Doing so with creativity, subtlety and grace is the art of narrative psychiatry.

## Notes

1. Marcia Linehan, *Cognitive-Behavioral Treatment of Borderline Personality Disorder* (New York: Guilford, 1993).
2. I engaged in a yearlong intensive narrative therapy training program at the Family Institute of Cambridge, taught by Sallyann Roth, Hugo Kamya, and Timothy Scott, in 1998–99.
3. Michael White, *"Re-authoring Conversations"* (workshop presented at The Family Institute of New Jersey, Metuchen, NJ, 1997).
4. Dulwich Centre, "Companions on a Journey: An Exploration of an Alternative Community Mental Health Project," *Dulwich Centre Newsletter* 1 (1997): 2–36.

5. Irving Kirsch, *The Emperor's New Drugs: Exploding the Antidepressant Myth* (New York: Basic Books, 2010); Robert Whitaker, *Anatomy of an Epidemic: Magic Bullets, Psychiatric Drugs, and the Astonishing Rise of Mental Illness in America* (New York: Crown, 2010); Daniel Carlat, *Unhinged: The Trouble with Psychiatry—A Doctor's Revelations about a Profession in Crisis* (New York: Simon & Schuster, 2010).

6. Stephen Gaddis, "Repositioning Traditional Research: Centering Clients' Accounts in the Construction of Professional Therapy Knowledges," *International Journal of Narrative Therapy and Community Work* 2 (2004): 37–48; Dulwich Centre Publications, "Narrative Therapy and Research," *International Journal of Narrative Therapy and Community Work* 2 (2004): 29–36; Ncazelo Ncube, "The Journey of Healing: Using Narrative Therapy and Map-Making to Respond to Child-Abuse in South Africa," *International Journal of Narrative Therapy and Community Work* 1 (2010): 3–12; Jane Speedy, "Living a More Peopled Life: Definitional Ceremony as Inquiry into Psychotherapy 'Outcomes,'" *International Journal of Narrative Therapy and Community Work* 3 (2004): 43–53; Rudi Kronbichter, "Narrative Therapy with Boys Struggling with Anorexia," *International Journal of Narrative Therapy and Community Work* 4 (2004): 55–70.

7. Lynette Vromans and Robert Schweitzer, "Narrative Therapy for Adults with a Major Depressive Disorder: Improved Symptom and Interpersonal Outcomes," *Psychotherapy Research* 21 (2010): 4–15; Mim Weber, Kierrynn Davis, and Lisa McPhie, "Narrative Therapy, Eating Disorders and Groups: Enhancing Outcomes in Rural NSW," *Australian Social Work* 59 (2006): 391–405; David Besa, "Evaluating Narrative Family Therapy using Single-System Research Designs," *Research on Social Work Practice* 4 (1994): 309–25.

8. For example, David Denborough of Dulwich Centre, Adelaide, Australia, in collaboration with John Henley and Julie Robinson of Flinders University, Adelaide, Australia, is studying the efficacy of the "Tree of Life" narrative approach to responding to vulnerable children; John Stillman, MSW, at Kenwood Therapy Center in Minnesota, USA, in collaboration with Christopher Erbes, PhD, at the University of Minnesota and the Veterans Affairs Medical Center, USA, are developing narrative treatment guidelines and studying efficacy of narrative approaches in the treatment of trauma; Laura Béres of Kings University College, London, Ontario, and Jim Duvall at the Hincks-Dellcrest Institute, Toronto, Ontario, with consultation from David Epston, are studying the effects of narrative therapy on both patients and therapists, including a focus on process and pivotal moments. From Dulwich Centre, "Research, Evidence, and Narrative Practice," accessed January 11, 2013, http://www.dulwichcentre.com.au/narrative-therapy-research.html.

9. Kathie Crocket et al., "Working for Ethical Research in Practice," *International Journal of Narrative Therapy and Community Work* 3 (2004): 61–66; Andrew Tootell, "Decentring Research Practice," *International Journal of Narrative Therapy and Community Work* 3 (2004): 54–55.

10. Michel Foucault, *Discipline and Punish: The Birth of the Prison*, trans. Alan Sheridan (New York: Random House, 1979); Michel Foucault, *The History of Sexuality, Volume I: An Introduction*, trans. Robert Hurley (New York: Random House, 1978).

11. Robin Morgan, ed., *Sisterhood Is Powerful* (New York: Random House, 1970); Virginia Woolf, *A Room of One's Own* (New York and London: Harcourt Brace Jovanovich, 1929); Alice Walker, *In Search of Our Mothers' Gardens* (New York: Harcourt, 1984).

12. Over the years, I have had the privilege of studying with Michael White, David Epston, Sallyann Roth, Shona Russell, Gaye Stockell, and Peggy Sax, among others.

13. Jill Freedman and Gene Combs, *Narrative Therapy: The Social Construction of Preferred Realities* (New York: W.W. Norton, 1996).
14. Gene Combs, personal communication, 2004.
15. SuEllen Hamkins, "Introducing Narrative Psychiatry: Narrative Approaches to Initial Psychiatric Consultations," *The International Journal of Narrative Therapy and Community Work* 1 (2005): 5–17; SuEllen Hamkins, "Bringing Narrative Practices to Psychopharmacology," *The International Journal of Narrative Therapy and Community Work* 1 (2010): 56–71.
16. Lewis Mehl-Madrona, *Healing the Mind through the Power of Story: The Promise of Narrative Psychiatry* (Rochester, VT: Bear, 2010).
17. Bradley Lewis, *Narrative Psychiatry: How Stories Can Shape Clinical Practice* (Baltimore, MD: Johns Hopkins University Press, 2011).
18. Please see Lewis, *Narrative Psychiatry,* 33–74, and Mehl-Madrona, *Healing the Mind,* 47–58 and 70–79, for more detailed descriptions of the theoretical origins of narrative psychiatry.
19. Michel Foucault, *The History of Madness*, ed. Jean Khalfa, trans. Jonathan Murphy (Abingdon, UK: Routledge, 2006); Foucault, *Discipline and Punish, History of Sexuality.*
20. Paul Ricoeur, *From Text to Action: Essays in Hermeneutics, II*, trans. Kathleen Blamey and John B. Thompson (Evanston, IL: Northwestern University Press, 1991).
21. Lewis, B., personal communication, 2012.
22. Barbara Myerhoff, *Number Our Days* (New York: Touchstone, 1979); Richard Schechter, *Essays in Performance Theory* (New York: Ralph Pine, for Drama School Specialists, 1977).
23. Michael White and David Epston, *Narrative Means to Therapeutic Ends* (New York: W.W. Norton, 1990).
24. Morgan, *Sisterhood Is Powerful*; Claudia Dreyfuss, ed., *Seizing Our Bodies: The Politics of Women's Health* (New York: Vintage, 1977); Adrienne Rich, *Blood, Bread and Poetry: Selected Prose 1979–1985* (New York: W.W. Norton, 1986); Alice Walker, *In Search of Our Mother's Gardens* (New York: Harcourt Brace Jovanovich, 1984).
25. Rita Charon, *Narrative Medicine: Honoring Stories of Illness* (New York: Oxford University Press, 2006).
26. Mehl-Madrona, *Healing the Mind*; Freeman and Combs, *Narrative Therapy*; Hamkins, "Narrative Psychiatry," "Narrative Approaches to Psychopharmacology."
27. Charon, *Narrative Medicine.*
28. Michael White, "Re-engaging with History: The Absent but Implicit," in *Reflections on Narrative Practice: Essays and Interviews*, ed. Michael White (Adelaide, Australia: Dulwich Centre Publications, 2000), 35.
29. "Patient," *Oxford English Dictionary,* accessed January 20, 2013, http://www.oed.com.silk.library.umass.edu/view/Entry/138820?rskey=D8n3FP&result=1&isAdvanced=false#eid

# PART ONE

# Foundations of
# Narrative Psychiatry

# CHAPTER ONE

# What Is Narrative Psychiatry?

Narrative psychiatry brings the muscle and agility of narrative theory and the spirit of compassion and social justice to the practice of psychiatry. What makes narrative psychiatry different from psychiatry-as-usual? Rather than focusing only on finding the source of the problem, narrative psychiatry also focuses on finding sources of strength and meaning. The result is compassionate, powerful healing.

Narrative psychiatry combines narrative and biological understandings of human suffering and well-being. It begins with compassionate connection with patients, understanding that we live our lives in relationships and connect with one another through the stories we tell. It relishes discovering untold but inspiring stories of a person's resiliency and skill in resisting mental health challenges while dismantling narratives that fuel problems. It examines what the doctor's kit of psychiatry has to offer in light of the values and preferences of the person seeking consultation, authorizing the patient as the arbiter of what is helpful and what is not.

Psychiatry as a field is seeking a more positive and patient-centered approach, which narrative psychiatry exemplifies. In his address at the American Psychiatric Association's annual meeting on May 6, 2012, President-Elect Dilip Jeste, M.D., said that "'positive psychiatry'—a psychiatry that aims not just to reduce psychiatric symptoms but to help patients grow and flourish—is the future."[1] Likewise, in 2012 the U.S. Substance Abuse and Mental Health Services Administration called for a focus on "recovery" that includes collaborative and culturally sensitive care that seeks to honor the patient's values, self-determination, and pre-ferred relationships and to foster not just the absence of symptoms, but also well-being.[2] Narrative approaches to psychiatry, psychotherapy, and medicine have been burgeoning in the last decade, inspired by the wave of narrative theory that has progressively suffused philosophy, anthro-pology, literature, and the arts over the last fifty years[3]. Training programs and courses teaching narrative approaches to mental health treatment and to medicine are flourishing.[4]

This chapter offers an overview of narrative psychiatry. First I'll explain what *narrative* means and why it's important. Next, to show narrative psychiatry in action and give you a gestalt of what it is, I'll present my work with my patient Jimmy Newman over the course of a year, intro-ducing and explaining key narrative psychiatry concepts. Then in each of the subsequent five chapters, I will address one of these key practices in more depth.

## WHY NARRATIVE?

It is through stories that we make meaning of our experiences. One could say that stories are *how* we experience ourselves and the world. As psychiatrist and philosopher Bradley Lewis puts it, "The stories people tell about themselves not only describe their lives but also shape their lives."[5] The stories told about us and that we tell create the reality in which we live. We humans are meaning-making creatures. We are continuously cre-ating narratives about what is happening in the world and to us person-ally. That is, we are constructing stories that understand the events of our lives over time according to a theme or plot—according to the meanings we give those events.

Stories can be simple or complex. *It's a beautiful day* is a simple story that interprets the weather events over the course of the morning—blue skies, a fresh breeze, radiant sunshine—and gives them meaning. *Today's unseasonably warm weather is evidence of the influence of human activ-ity on the planet* is a more complex story that looks at the events of the morning's temperature, historic weather patterns, and the production of carbon dioxide over time and links them according to the theme of global warming. These stories influence how we experience the blue skies and radiant sunshine, and they influence our actions: Do I stay inside or go out? Do I drive to the farmers' market or ride my bike?

Stories are based on what we value. They are not arbitrary. That there are multiple stories about the same events does not mean that every story is equally valid—in fact, it means the opposite. Different stories arise because events that occur are valued differently by different people. Any story can be queried to determine what values it is based on, and understanding those values gives us the basis for deciding how "true" the story is.

Focusing on the narratives of our lives makes them more visible. For example, I would invite you to pause and consider the story of the journey that brought you to read this book. If you could turn to another reader and tell the story of that journey, what would you say? What does that journey say about what you value?

Our identities are constituted in the meanings we give the events in our lives—in what we value. That is, our identities are based on the stories we tell about ourselves, stories such as, *I am a psychotherapist. I am a fiddle player. I am a success. I am a failure.* When patients are suffering emotionally, the meanings they give to the events of their lives often follow themes of personal failure, regret, unworthiness, pointlessness, isolation, and so on, themes that can increase their suffering and foster an impoverished sense of who they are. Cultivating narratives that honor our patients' integrity and resourcefulness despite their duress—that offer alternative plot lines to the stories of their lives—can bring energy, inspiration, clarity, hope, direction, companionship, and emotional relief. That is, these new stories can be healing.

What we can know and remember about ourselves and the world depends on its inclusion in a narrative.[6] Prominent narrative philosopher Paul Ricoeur writes, "Human action is an open work, the meaning of which is 'in suspense.'"[7] The meaning we give an action ushers it into a particular story with particular consequences: *Last week I missed a day of work; I am on the road to failure, I might as well give up. Last week, I went to work four days; I am on the road to success, I can keep going.*

Our intentions arise from what we give meaning and our intentions mold our actions. Jerome Bruner, a cognitive psychologist whose work informs narrative psychiatry, writes, "The central concept of a human psychology is *meaning* and processes and transactions involved in the construction of meanings."[8] He resists understanding human nature "as nothing but the concatenation of conditioned reflexes, associative bonds, transformed animal drives."[9] Bruner emphasizes how our intentions are a paramount force in determining how we experience ourselves and what we do. When we help our patients clarify their values and intentions, they develop a fresh sense of what might be possible for their lives.

### Narrative Ideas That Inform Narrative Psychiatry

We make meaning and become who we are through our relationships in the context of our culture.

Stories are how we make meaning of our experiences.

The stories told about us and that we tell shape our experience of reality.

Our identities are constituted in the narratives we tell about the events in our lives and in what we value.

Nascent stories of strength and meaning can be cultivated into narratives that are resources for recovery.

What we value gives rise to our intentions, which guide our actions.

Cultural narratives and practices that share common values give rise to discourses that can have powerful effects, yet may remain largely invisible.

The discourses that influence us can be deconstructed to reveal the values on which they are based.

Discourses that fuel problems can be countered, and narratives and practices that are life enhancing can be nurtured.

We make meaning and become who we are through our relationships in the context of our culture. Meaning making and storytelling are social phenomena. We negotiate our identities in relation to the narratives that others hold about us, those close to us as well as discourses in the wider culture. *Discourses* are narratives and practices that share common values. Often wider cultural discourses are invisible as such and are taken as common sense. Discourses include expectations, stories, standards, customs, laws, and so on that have real effects on our lives: *You are a success and can join our group. You are a failure and cannot join our group.* Narrative psychiatry seeks to identify and understand the discourses that are affecting our patients. In doing so, discourses that fuel problems can be countered and stories and practices that are life enhancing can be nurtured.

When I first learned these key narrative ideas in my intensive course on narrative therapy at what was then The Family Institute of Cambridge back in 1998, I was excited and intimidated. Excited because the ideas rang true, promoted awareness of social issues, and were intellectually beautiful; intimidated because they were completely foreign to how I had been trained as a psychiatrist and psychotherapist. The turning point for me occurred in a conversation I had with a psychologist who, like me, had been initially trained in psychodynamic psychotherapy. We realized that we had been attending to our patients' narratives all along, but now, instead of primarily uncovering stories of what was painful or conflicted in their lives, we could use our psychotherapeutic skills to uncover stories of what was sustaining and inspiring.

## KEY PRACTICES OF NARRATIVE PSYCHIATRY: JIMMY'S STORY

I first met Jimmy Newman as he was beginning his first year of college. Jimmy had distinguished himself in high school as a student and an athlete, and had been looking forward to college to continue those successes. A month earlier, in August, a few days after using marijuana and LSD, Jimmy had developed a severe manic episode, his first, during which he became agitated and delusional, was hospitalized for five days, was treated with lithium and the antipsychotic aripiprazole, completed a three-week partial hospitalization program, and then a week later went to college. I was to be his new psychiatrist, working with him in conjunction with one of the psychotherapists at our counseling center. She had already met with him and had apprised me that Jimmy had had a mild recurrence of manic symptoms over his second weekend at college in the context of stopping his medicine and engaging in drug use.

At our first meeting, as he sat stiffly on the edge of the couch in my office, Jimmy was composed, but somber, apprehensive, and reticent. A compact, muscular eighteen-year-old European American man, Jimmy simultaneously exuded tenacity and vulnerability.

How did narrative psychiatry guide me in working with Jimmy?

My first task as a narrative psychiatrist was to form a connection with him that respected who he was and where he was emotionally. In this, I hoped to create a collaborative therapeutic alliance in which Jimmy felt seen and heard. Second, I wanted to hear and strengthen the story of who Jimmy was without the problem,[10] and what his vision was for his life—that is, his preferred identity. In narrative psychiatry, *preferred identity* is what one values most about who one is and who one might become. In Jimmy's case, I was particularly sensitive to the fact that the story of his preferred identity as a successful student and athlete was at risk of being overshadowed by a story of identity that emphasized mental illness. Third, I wanted to hear his experience of the problem and come to a common understanding of its nature, speaking about the problem as separate from, or external to, who he was as a person. Fourth, I wished to determine how he was succeeding in mitigating the problem, thereby creating a story with the theme of success in facing a difficult problem. My hope was to actively develop and extend this story of success with further detail, additional examples over time, connection with important people in his life, and opportunities to share and retell it. Last, in collaboration with Jimmy, I intended to examine what next steps he wanted to take and what psychiatric resources, such as medicine and psychotherapy, might be helpful. Over the months of working together, I hoped to continue the process of connecting, developing stories of preferred identity, understanding the nature of the problem, developing narratives of strength and meaning, refining the use of psychiatric resources, taking steps to support his vision of well-being, and reflecting on what was helpful.

---

**Key Practices of Narrative Psychiatry**

Foster empathic attunement and collaborative connection

Start with stories of success:
    —seeing the person without the problem

Understand the patient's experience of the problem:
    —seeing the problem as external to the person

Develop stories of strength and meaning and deconstruct narratives that fuel problems:
    —attending to values and intentionality

Collaboratively consider psychiatric resources in light of the patient's values

Support the patient in taking steps toward his or her vision of wellbeing

---

## CONNECTING WITH STRENGTHS

In our first meeting, I focused first on connection—just as I would have before practicing narrative psychiatry. I wanted Jimmy to feel that I could see and hear and feel his fortitude as well as his worry. I began by engaging with him in an area of strength, asking him about school and what he was thinking of majoring in. Our conversation went something like this:

S:  Have you thought about what you might major in?

JIMMY:  Environmental science.

S:  What interests you about environmental science?

JIMMY:  (Shrugs.)

I switched to a different area that he might feel more positive about.

S:   I hear that you run cross-country.
JIMMY:   (Nods.)
S:   And will you be running at college?
JIMMY:   Yeah. It's just a club sport here though.
S:   I see. And have practices started yet?
JIMMY:   No.
S:   What do you like about running?
JIMMY:   (Shrugs, but looks interested.)
S:   Did you enjoy running in high school?
JIMMY:   (With a hint of pride and pleasure, but mostly modesty.) Yeah.
S:   You pretty good at it?
JIMMY:   Good enough.

I was connecting here with the Jimmy who is an athlete, but who is also modest and not one to brag. (I found out after our appointment that he was one of the high school state champions.) In my attention to who he was, in my close listening to the emotional tone of his responses, we were forging a therapeutic alliance in which he felt seen and heard *and* we were simultaneously strengthening the story of his identity as an athlete. In narrative psychiatry, our nuanced awareness of our patients' narratives is both a way to connect with and understand them and a way to strengthen stories that are healing. Narrative psychiatry continuously attends to the narrative of a person's identity, seeking to develop the story of who the person is without the problem. In Jimmy's case, I probed to get a sense of what aspect of his identity he felt good about sharing with me. He was lukewarm about academics, but more eager to share his story as a runner. I wanted the story of his success as an athlete to take precedence over the story of his mental health challenges in his narrative of who he is.

In my work with Jimmy, I was implicitly attending to the stories that are in circulation about people who have had psychiatric hospitalizations. In my development as a narrative practitioner, I learned to pay

**Questions to Understand the Person without the Problem**

What are your sources of inspiration?
When do you feel most alive?
What aspects of life do you find most fulfilling?
What do you love to do?
What is bringing you the most interest and pleasure these days?
What vision might you have for your life?

attention to the wider cultural stories about narratives like Jimmy's, to the meta-narratives that impact patients. I am aware that there are powerful social discourses that denigrate the identity of those who experience bipolar symptoms and make negative conclusions about their characters, abilities, and prospects. I wanted to minimize the power of those discourses to influence Jimmy's creation of his identity at a time when, as a young adult, he was just beginning to clarify who he was and what he cared about.

## UNDERSTANDING THE PATIENT'S STORY ABOUT THE PROBLEM

In addition to honoring Jimmy's strengths, I wanted to honor how hard the mental health challenges that he faced have been, to further our empathic connection and to make room for the story of his experience.

S: So you've really been through something? With the hospitalization and everything?
Jimmy: (Shrugs.)
S: How was that for you?
Jimmy: (Shrugs.)
S: Not how you wanted to spend your last month before college?

JIMMY:  (Shakes his head.)

S:  Pretty much of a drag, huh?

JIMMY:  (Nods.)

S:  What helped you get through all that?

JIMMY:  (Shrugs.)

It was clear that Jimmy was not finding it timely to share the story of his experience of being hospitalized. On an emotional level, I could feel his grief, his desire to not get emotional, and his appreciation that I seemed to get what he had gone through. I didn't press him to say more. Rather, I became practical and reviewed with him what I knew from the hospital discharge summary, asking him his opinion of the accuracy of the report. He was attentive and made brief replies to my questions. He agreed with the doctor's description of his symptoms of agitation and grandiose delusions. My sharing the report with him and asking him to evaluate it empowered him as the authority on his experience, implicitly supported his agency and knowledge, and helped foster a collaborative therapeutic alliance.

A diagnosis is a story. Like any story, it is told from a particular perspective based on particular values. The story that a person has bipolar disorder is a psychiatric one that emphasizes the ways in which genetic predisposition, stress, and brain chemistry can lead to symptoms of depression or mania, and that shows how medicine can be an important resource, along with adequate sleep, in preventing symptoms. Bipolar disorder has been a hot topic recently, with concerns raised about the dramatic increase in the number of children who have been diagnosed in the last decade.[11] Because of this, particular discernment is needed to determine whether the diagnosis is a useful narrative for understanding a person's experience, with care to neither over- nor underattribute symptoms to that diagnosis. In other words, it can be as unhelpful to ignore the possibility that bipolar disorder is present as it is to overdiagnose it. In this, narrative psychiatry is interested in thoughtfully considering the narratives influencing our understanding of bipolar disorder, with care to honor the values and perspectives of the patients.

I asked Jimmy if he agreed with the diagnosis the doctors in the hospital had made: bipolar disorder. He seemed a little surprised by the question and paused before answering. He said he could see why they made the diagnosis, but he remained hopeful that his symptoms of mania just occurred because of his drug use, and that he didn't have bipolar disorder.

In Jimmy's case, he and I shared the hope that his symptoms had been triggered by his drug use and might not recur if he abstained, meaning that he might not have bipolar disorder. At the same time, we shared the realization that his symptoms had been particularly severe, that they came back when he stopped his medicine for a few days, and that he might indeed have bipolar disorder. His overarching value was that he wanted to have a successful first year at college and wanted to be sure that symptoms of mania would not interfere with that. We had come to a common understanding of the nature of the problem, including that the problem might change over time.

## COAUTHORING NEW NARRATIVES OF STRENGTH AND MEANING

Medicine, while at times helpful, is never the reason why someone is succeeding in pursuing their dreams. That success is due to the person's intentions, values, talents, commitments, creativity, and tenacity—and our job as narrative psychiatrists is making sure that story of success is told. In focusing on cultivating stories of patients' strengths and values, narrative psychiatry departs from psychiatry as it is usually practiced. When I first tried to do so years ago, it felt unfamiliar and awkward; but as I developed as a narrative psychiatrist, my comfort and skill grew. As Jimmy and I began to speak about his success in overcoming mania, he told me that he decided to stop using drugs like marijuana and LSD so he could stay well, and he was willing to continue the lithium and aripiprazole, as it seemed symptoms might come back if he didn't. While mood stabilizers seemed to be an important part of his success in constraining the problem, I was also interested in developing a story of success that was more intimately linked to who he was a person. In other words, while the medicine might be providing him with support, it was not the reason why he was able to have a successful start at college.

To become part of an ongoing narrative of identity—to "stick"—a new story needs to be compelling. It can't be based on just one event of a person's life. Rather, it needs to link multiple events together over time according to a theme; in our case, a theme of success. The things that make for a good story in narrative psychiatry are the same things that make for a good story in literature: lush sensory detail, an emotionally engaging plot, and characters we care about. The other thing that makes a new story compelling is for it to be told and retold. Stories are strengthened by being in circulation.

Here is how I developed the story of Jimmy's success in overcoming the problem of mania and pursuing his intention of succeeding at college:

S:  Getting hospitalized and doing the partial hospitalization program in August, and then coming to your first semester of college in September—I just want to pause and notice that it takes something to be able to do that.

JIMMY:  (shrugs.)

S:  Overcoming a challenge like the one you faced and continuing right on with your plan to come to college, I imagine that takes determination, would you agree?

JIMMY:  I guess.

S:  Is that a good word for it, determination?

JIMMY:  Yes.

S:  Do you have a sense of where this determination comes from? Is it something new, or have you had determination in the past?

JIMMY:  Ummm, well, I would say I developed it running cross-country.

S:  You competed all through high school, is that right?

JIMMY:  Yeah.

S:  And did you use determination like, within a race, to win it, or was it determination to practice hard?

JIMMY:  It was both. I worked hard toward what I wanted to achieve, in practices and in races.

S:  And would you say that that the determination to work hard toward what you want to achieve helped you overcome the symptoms you faced in August and be able to come to college?

JIMMY:  Yes, I would say it did.

S:  And how is college going?

JIMMY:  (Shrugs.) It's hard. My classes are really challenging. The concepts are harder; it's not like high school.

S:  No, it's not like high school. How's it going doing the homework?

JIMMY:  I'm getting it done. I wrote an essay for a class and I went to the writing center to get help on it, which is not something I have usually done. But I'll do whatever it takes.

S:  So academically, you're using determination and doing whatever it takes to succeed, like going to the writing center and doing your homework. And how is the other part of college going, making connections?

JIMMY:  Good. I've made some new friends, and I hang out with some old friends, too.

S:  Now, you said that you have stopped doing drugs so that you can stay well, but I imagine perhaps some of your old friends still are using.

JIMMY:  Yes, but I'm not going to. I turned down free marijuana for the first time last week.

S:  Wow, I imagine that took a kind of determination.

JIMMY:  Yes it did, but I am committed to not using drugs.

S:  This commitment of yours, to work hard to achieve your goals, to do whatever it takes, are there roots of that in your family, would you say?

JIMMY:  I dunno.

S:  Did your parents ever have to work hard to overcome difficulty?

JIMMY:  Yes. They are both very hardworking.

S: So, would you say you got some of your determination to do whatever it takes from them?

JIMMY: Yes, I guess it's genetic. (Smiles.)

You can hear in this conversation how I first sought a name for a new theme of success in coming to college. Jimmy didn't offer one, so I posed the possibility that *determination* would be a way to understand his efforts in coming to college, and I checked it out with him to see if he agreed that it is a fit. It might not have been, he might have disagreed, and then I would have offered other words or phrases to characterize his success. *Determination* is a valued and validating aspect of Jimmy's identity that represents an aspect of his character. It is a strength of his, and naming it makes it more available for him to draw on.

### Sample Questions to Elicit Stories about a Person's Strengths

What does your ability to persevere in that way say about your capabilities?

Would *creativity* be a word that might describe your approach to that problem?

What did you draw on to be able to succeed in that way?

What name might you give to this ability of yours?

What would you say it took to be able to overcome that problem?

Valued personal qualities and strengths, such as determination, are harnessed in the service of the person's intentions. Aspects of character or elements of a person's nature are experienced as desirable or undesirable to the extent that they contribute to or detract from a person's vision for his life. Richer and more compelling narratives that honor our patients' agency arise from exploring how their intentions, values, and vision have contributed to their success, as opposed to understanding success only in terms of character traits, which if considered exclusively can contribute to a sense of inevitability and a lack of agency.[12] Therefore, whenever we identify strengths or personal resources, we can honor our patients' identities and agency, and add vibrant color, movement, and initiative by eliciting stories of how these personal qualities contribute to the person's *intentions* for creating the life he or she wants to be living.

As Jimmy and I spoke about determination, he made statements about his efforts to manifest his intentions (*I worked hard toward what I want to achieve, But I'll do whatever it takes*), adding agency and specificity to the story of his success. Repeating his words creates a more personally compelling and vivid narrative. I traced the history of Jimmy's determination to work hard toward what he wants to achieve and to do whatever it takes across time and across different aspects of his life: running, doing college work, resisting drugs. I could have further strengthened these stories by asking for more details, such as asking for the story of a specific tournament in which determination played an important role: *Where was the race? Who was it against? What was the course like? Who was watching? Which moment of the race stands out to you?* Likewise, I could have enriched these narratives by asking Jimmy to say more about the meaning of working hard toward what he wants to achieve and doing whatever it takes in his life: *Tell me more about what it is that you want to achieve. Is what you want to achieve linked to larger commitments you have in your life? You will do whatever it takes in service of what vision for your life? What is it like for you to see yourself do whatever it takes?* I didn't do so at that time because Jimmy was so reticent in our meeting that I worried he would have felt badgered by such questions.

I then linked Jimmy's story to important people in his life; in this case, he identified his parents as the source of his determination to do whatever it takes to succeed. I particularly like his statement that this commitment was genetic. It stands in powerful contrast to the usual focus of family history when bipolar disorder is being considered as a diagnosis. It's not that knowing genetic vulnerability to bipolar disorder isn't important; it's just not the only thing that is important. Family strengths, genetic or not, are a critical resource in overcoming mental health

**Sample Questions to Elicit Stories about a Person's Intentions, Values, and Vision**

Toward what goal are you harnessing your capability to persevere?
What vision for your life are you hoping to achieve?
What does your effort to succeed in that way say about your intentions for your life?
Is your skill of friendliness linked to a value you hold?
Is what you did evidence of commitments you have for how you live your life?

challenges, and they become more available to our patients when we highlight them through stories.

## CONSIDERING PSYCHIATRIC RESOURCES IN LIGHT OF THE PATIENT'S VALUES

Next Jimmy and I addressed which psychiatric resources might be most helpful to him. He was willing to take lithium and aripiprazole for the present, although he wanted to stop them as soon as possible. He wondered if the aripiprazole, at a dose of 10 mg daily, was causing him to feel a bit emotionally shut down. He noted that he is usually energetic and outgoing, and he was not feeling as much that way currently. We discussed the pros and cons of medication use, such as the recurrence of symptoms when he stopped them; the kindling effect, in which each episode of mania makes the person more vulnerable to subsequent episodes; the risks of lithium to his kidneys; and the risk of weight gain and metabolic syndrome from the aripiprazole. We made a collaborative plan to continue the medicines unchanged for the present, to check his lithium level, and to begin a slow taper of the aripiprazole later in the semester if everything was going well. He was happy to continue to see his psychotherapist. We discussed the importance of sleep, healthy diet, and hydration. While Jimmy was committed to giving up drugs, he did plan on engaging in moderate alcohol use as part of what he valued about the college experience, and we discussed ways to minimize his risks in doing so, ultimately coming up with the plan that he would combine his vodka with Gatorade to prevent dehydration.

## SUPPORTING THE PATIENT IN TAKING STEPS TOWARD HIS VISION OF WELL-BEING

Near the end of our initial meeting, I asked Jimmy if he would like me to bring his parents into our conversation. Of course I would have respected his preferences either way, but I asked for two reasons: first, because young adults who have had manic episodes can benefit from the involvement of their parents or other caring adults in their treatment; and second, so I could strengthen the stories of Jimmy's success. He granted permission readily, and I rang up his mother right there in the session. Calling her in his presence honored his authority and gave transparency to the nature of the call. I shared the story of Jimmy's determination to succeed at school and to do whatever it takes to stay on course, emphasizing the challenge it is to start college right after a psychiatric hospitalization, and strengthening this story of success by repeating it and widening its circulation. This also set the stage for understanding that it wouldn't be surprising if he did have new symptoms, and that we could adjust our treatment plan accordingly. His mother readily agreed with the story that Jimmy is one to do whatever it takes to succeed, and was pleased that he linked that ability with his family genetic inheritance. We discussed issues of diagnosis and treatment, and I encouraged her to call me with any questions or concerns.

Jimmy had created a plan for manifesting his vision of creating a successful first year of college. Drawing on his determination to do whatever it took to succeed, he was using resources such as the writing center to support his academic success, and he was creating friendships and developing as an athlete through running. He made choices to avoid illicit drugs, to take psychotropic medication, to engage in psychotherapy, and to welcome the support of his family.

And that concluded Jimmy's and my fifty-minute initial appointment.

## A YEAR OF NARRATIVE PSYCHIATRY

Over the course of the semester, Jimmy and I met for twenty minutes every other week, and he met with his psychotherapist weekly, who continued to develop narratives of who he was and what was helping him succeed. If I had been the primary psychotherapist, I would have seen Jimmy weekly for fifty minutes and done the same. Whether we are primary psychotherapists or psychiatrists working in collaboration with a psychotherapist, we have a particularly important role in supporting positive identity development and resilience because it is our responsibility to understand the meaning of our patients' symptoms and experiences—that is, the story of who they are and the diagnosis that fits their problems. We have been imbued by our culture with authority by virtue of being licensed professionals who are considered to have expertise in such matters. Working collaboratively and transparently helps to mitigate the power differential inherent in the treatment relationship. For psychiatrists or psychiatric nurse practitioners, even when our primary role is as diagnostician and psychopharmacologist, we are always also psychotherapists—that is, we are endeavoring to engage with our patients in ways that are psychologically therapeutic. Narrative psychiatry offers us particularly helpful tools to do so. Irrespective of what kind of psychotherapy our patients are simultaneously engaged in, narrative approaches to psychiatric consultation are complementary and are experienced by them as supportive and healing.

A month into the semester, Jimmy developed symptoms of depression, with negative thoughts, not enjoying things, and not wanting to see his friends, and was sleeping twelve hours a day. He remained hopeful, but felt very tired, and sometimes fell asleep in class. He remained committed to pull through, drawing on his commitment to do whatever it takes, and connecting with his friends, family, and psychotherapist. He also wanted us to consider reducing the aripiprazole because he felt it was making him tired. After considering all the pros and cons, he elected to taper the aripiprazole down to 5 mg daily. I wasn't sure if this would help or hurt his depression, but it was his strong preference to decrease the aripiprazole, so that is what we tried first. Five days later he was feeling much better: less tired and less depressed.

Racing season started, and he was a leader in that arena. He made new friends at college and pulled away a bit from his high school friends who were still using drugs. He let his new friends know he was using lithium. He kept up with his coursework. At the end of the semester, we began to slowly decrease the aripiprazole further and he successfully tapered off of it over the winter without a recurrence of symptoms. He became more animated in our meetings.

In the second semester he asked to go off of the lithium. We spoke at length about the pros and cons. He was happy that he had a successful adjustment to college, was doing well in his classes, and made friends with guys on the cross-country team, with whom he was planning on getting an apartment for his sophomore year. I always keep in mind when speaking with people about their medicine that, in the privacy of their own homes, they have complete freedom to take it or not. While I may be the expert about the medicine and its effects, the patient is the expert on his or her life. Any medication decisions will be based on what that person values. Jimmy valued his success at college and said he could see why it might make sense to continue the lithium, but ultimately he decided to begin to reduce the lithium during the semester and then to go off of it completely over the summer, under the care of his psychiatrist from home. His value was that one episode of mania was not enough to warrant a lifetime use of lithium.

When I saw him again in the middle of August, he reported he was feeling well, sleeping well, and looking forward to starting his second year of college. We made a plan for how he would get help should symptoms recur. He told all his apartment mates what he was doing, and instructed them to call his parents should he start to appear overenergized or otherwise not himself. I spoke with his parents as well.

I had last seen Jimmy a week before writing this chapter and he was doing well. He felt like he was back to his usual outgoing, active self. We celebrated his successes, and he agreed to check in with me monthly and to call with any questions or concerns between appointments. We discussed the signs of symptom recurrence, and I asked him what he would do should that happen. "I'll just go back on the lithium. If I need it, I need it. It's not that big of a deal to me." This really moved me. He wasn't in denial about the possibility that it might turn out that he had bipolar disorder, but it clearly wasn't the defining feature of his identity.

I don't know that our conversations about his stance of doing whatever it took to succeed, our honoring of his genetic legacy of determination in the service of his vision for his life, my respect for his choices about alcohol, or our collaboration in making medication decisions made the difference in his success at overcoming a mental health challenge, developing a positive identity, and thriving in college. I am clear, however, that the practices of narrative psychiatry I employed are designed to help in just these ways, and that it was inspiring for me to see and hear Jimmy's stories of success.

Toward the end of that appointment, I asked him permission to use his story for this book, and he agreed, choosing the name Jimmy for his pseudonym. I asked him, "So would you say that dealing with the hospitalization and taking lithium and everything, was that one of the hardest things you've had to do in your life?"

"Oh, no," he said. "Practicing for cross-country, the long workouts and the races and everything, that was way harder than this."

## Notes

1. American Psychiatric Association, "Ingredients of Successful Aging Exist Now, Says APA President-Elect," *Psychiatric News Update* 19 (2012),.
2. Substance Abuse and Mental Health Services Administration, "SAMHSA's Working Definition of Recovery from Mental Disorders and Substance Use Disorders," *SAMHSA Blog*, December 22, 2011, http://blog.samhsa.gov/2011/12/22/samhsa%E2%80%99s-definition-and-guiding-principles-of-recovery-%E2%80%93-answering-the-call-for-feedback/.

3. Foucault, *Discipline and Punish*; Schechter, *Performance Theory*; Jerome Bruner, *Acts of Meaning* (Cambridge, MA: Harvard University Press, 1990); Lewis, *Narrative Psychiatry*; Mehl-Madrona, *Healing the Mind*; Michael White, *Maps of Narrative Practice* (New York: W.W. Norton, 2007); Charon, *Narrative Medicine*.

4. For example: The Dulwich Centre, Adelaide, Australia, www.dulwichcentre.com.au; Narrative Practices Adelaide, Adelaide, Australia, led by Maggie Carey, Shona Russell, Rob Hall, and Lisa Johnson, http://www.narrativepractices.com.au/; The Evanston Family Therapy Center, Evanston, Illinois, led by Jill Freedman and Gene Combs, www.narrativetherapychicago.com; Family Therapy Training Boston, Boston, Massachusetts, with Corky Becker, http://www.familytherapytrainingboston.com/; The Kenwood Center, Minneapolis, Minnesota, led by Walter Bera, http://www.kenwoodcenter.org/therapy/about.html; The Narrative Practice and Collaborative Inquiry Study Group, Vermont, led by Peggy Sax, http://reauthoringteaching.com/npci_consultation_group.html; The Vancouver School for Narrative Therapy, led by Stephen Madigan, http://therapeuticconversations.com/; Family Centered Services Project, Watertown, Massachusetts, led by William Madsen, http://www.family-centeredservices.org/; David Epston, New Zealand, http://www.narrativeapproaches.com/Training%20Folder/narrative_training.htm; Bay Area Family Therapy Training Associates, Cupertino, California, led by Jeffrey Zimmerman, http://www.baftta.com/; The Narrative Therapy Centre of Toronto, led by Angel Yuen, Maisa-Said Albis, and Ruth Pluznick, http://www.narrativetherapycentre.com; The Narrative Therapy Initiative at the Salem Center, Salem, Massachusetts, led by Stephen Gaddis, http://narrativetherapyinitiative.wikispaces.com/Narrative+Therapy+Classes; the Program in Narrative Medicine, Columbia University, New York, http://www.cumc.columbia.edu/dept/medicine/narrativemed/writing.html; and Institute for Dialogic Practice, Haydenville, Massachusetts, led by Mary Olsen, http://www.dialogicpractice.net/ .

5. Lewis, *Narrative Psychiatry*, 66.

6. Bruner, *Acts of Meaning*, 56.

7. Ricoeur, *From Text to Action*, 155.

8. Bruner, *Acts of Meaning*, 33.

9. Bruner, *Acts of Meaning*, 31.

10. Michael White wrote, "The person is not the problem…the problem is the problem." Michael White, *Selected Papers* (Adelaide, Australia: Dulwich Centre Publications, 1989), 52.

11. Carlat, *Unhinged*, 145; Whitaker, *Anatomy of an Epidemic*, 172–204.

12. Michael White, *Maps of Narrative Practice* (New York: W.W. Norton, 2007), 104–5.

# CHAPTER TWO

# Connecting with Compassion

*The Therapeutic Relationship*

Compassionate connection is the heart of narrative psychiatry. As humans, we live our lives in relationships. Who we are and what we feel—the very development of our nervous systems—arises through our connection and emotional resonance with others.[1] The quality of that attunement determines what is possible for us to feel and to know of ourselves. The meanings we give our experiences and feelings—the stories we tell about who we are—arise in relationships. Every story has a teller and an audience, and the nature of that audience determines what kind of story it is possible to tell. Telling an emotionally moving story in a way that is healing requires an empathically attuned listener. For all these reasons, connecting with our patients is our first priority.

Creating a therapeutic alliance with our patients begins with emotional attunement and is strengthened by transparency and collaboration. That is, in narrative psychiatry, we are open with our patients about our thought processes and we work with them in a side-by-side stance to look together at the problems they are facing, the values and strengths they can develop, and the treatment resources they can choose to draw upon. Addressing the impact on patients' lives of racial, cultural, sexual, gender, and other identities and narratives with sensitivity to issues of privilege and oppression also builds trust. Attending thoughtfully to issues of power in the doctor-patient relationship serves to empower patients as partners in the treatment process. Supporting patients in developing empathic communities of support outside of therapy expands opportunities for healing connections in patients' lives. Let's look at how we can put these ideas into practice, starting with developing emotional attunement.

## EMOTIONAL ATTUNEMENT

Empathic emotional attunement is connection at its core, and from infancy on, experiencing another's empathic attunement is soothing to us, body and soul. It is, in itself, healing. Becoming emotionally attuned with someone means listening with your whole being. It is attending not only to what you see and hear, but also what you feel in your gut and in your heart in being with the other person, and responding compassionately from that place. Attunement requires us to attend simultaneously to the emotions arising in the other person and to the emotions arising in ourselves. Our awareness and acceptance of the feelings that are arising, our empathic resonance with another person, deepens and enriches our experience of connection and leads to greater and greater attunement.[2]

We manifest emotional attunement in all kinds of ways. In 1988, when I was a medical intern working on the neurology unit in a hospital in Cleveland, I was responsible for admitting and caring for an elderly woman I'll call Mrs. Eason, who had apparently had a stroke. (I've changed the identifying details of this story.) She was found collapsed downtown with $305 in cash in a bank envelope, her Blue Cross insurance card, and a card with the name of her mechanic, "Bob." I tried to be as reassuring as I could while completing her physical exam, gently telling her what I was doing, unsure what she could understand. Although awake and alert, she was weak on one side and was unable to speak or communicate with us in writing or any other way, so we had no idea how to contact her family. From the anguished, pleading look in her eyes, I could tell that she was terrified. I knew she needed loved ones to bring her comfort at this time, but her insurance company listed no next of kin, and there was no answer at her home phone when I called. Here is what I wrote in my journal at the time about caring for her:

> I call the service station. Bob tells me she is his 'play aunt' and gives me the name of his mother, her friend. "What? Addie Eason is in the hospital? With a stroke? No, she's never been sick. She is still working, in private homes now, house cleaning. She's widowed. Never had no children. And her own family never appreciated her."
>
> So that's it. A previously healthy 75-year-old Black woman has a stroke, and now cannot speak and cannot move her right arm. I go to her room where she is lying in bed. It's four-thirty. She is still. I know she cannot understand me. I say I know, I know, I know. I sit on the edge of the bed, put my arm around her, and rock her.
>
> The next day, she is very much the same—no speech, disoriented, weak. Again, between seeing eleven other patients, rounds, teaching, and preparing a talk, I sit for ten minutes rocking this woman who does not know where she is, nor who I am, nor what is happening.
>
> On her third day in the hospital, I see her with a physical therapist in the middle of the corridor where I am clustered with six other residents during rounds. She is walking! I am delighted. Then it happens. She sees me, and her eyes, those expressive eyes, light up and she raises her good hand and waves at me, at just me amid all those doctors, a tiny wave. She smiles radiantly. Her eyes say, I know.
>
> That smile was the feast that sustained me this week.

Speech was not necessary for our connection. In sitting with Mrs. Eason, I felt with her the enormity of her loss and her aloneness and responded with the comfort of my full presence. In rocking her, I conveyed my care and compassion in a language I felt sure she would understand. My attunement communicated to her that no matter what her state, I could join her there and would not abandon her. I could share her pain in having a stroke and her joy that she could still walk.

Every day, for the week that Mrs. Eason was on my service before transferring to a rehabilitation hospital, she grew stronger. When I saw her at her bedside each morning, though she could not speak, she grasped my hand in hers and shook it, looking at me with eyes that shone like lanterns, conveying gratitude, hope, fear, and relief. I gazed back at her, letting her know that I could be there with her. She could experience what she was feeling and know she was held in relationship. This is the first gift of emotional attunement.

Of course, rocking a patient is only rarely the most appropriate way to manifest attunement. Rocking was what I felt moved to do with Mrs. Eason, but each of us conveys our care for and attunement with our patients in ways that uniquely suit us. With Mrs. Eason, others of us may have taken her hand, spoken to her in soothing tones, or sat quietly for a moment at her bedside. Attunement is about the emotional resonance between oneself and one's patient, and what that looks like is particular to each of us and to each situation.

As a psychiatrist, when I meet with patients I try to attend carefully to the emotions that are arising in them and to the stream of emotions that are arising in me in resonance with them. What do I see and hear, what do I feel in my solar plexus, my chest, my face? Are tears rising in me, anger, fear, tenderness, playfulness, joy? When I can feel those feelings and observe that I am feeling those feelings, it is calming and clarifying to me, and, often, moving. From that place of equanimity and emotional resonance, I can convey my awareness and acceptance of these emotions to the patient in myriad ways, in my demeanor, the expression on my face, the tone of my voice, and in what I say. When I succeed, this emotional validation encourages my patients to feel what they are feeling more fully, to be more aware of what they are feeling, and to be more accepting of what they are feeling. This creates healing and connection, which patients communicate by becoming more relaxed, more forthcoming, more self-accepting, and more hopeful, often saying in words how helpful it is to feel understood and accepted.

## EMOTIONAL ATTUNEMENT AND HEALING NARRATIVES

The second gift of emotional attunement is that it makes it possible to speak about what is felt most deeply. To discover and nurture narratives that open up new possibilities for healing, a psychiatrist needs to see and hear and feel what is most meaningful to the patient and to have the patient feel heard and seen and felt. The quality of listening—the degree of attunement—determines what emotions are safe to feel and what stories are safe to tell. By *safe,* I mean feeling that one will continue to be held in an empathic relationship no matter what one feels or says. When her doctor is emotionally attuned with her, a patient knows she can speak of what is most precious to her and have it be received with compassion. She can tell an emotionally moving story in a way that is healing; that is, in a way that brings forward new understandings of who she is and what might be possible for her life.

Attuning to joy is just as important as attuning to sorrow. Anne Rabinowitz came to see me last week for her usual every-two-month appointment. A 51-year-old Jewish woman of European American ancestry, Anne worked full-time to support herself and enjoyed traveling with her sister to the ocean in the summer. She had successfully vanquished severe mood symptoms that had disrupted her life for several decades. In the past, she had utilized psychiatric hospitalizations on several occasions to help her through times when it wasn't clear to her that life was worth living. She found her medications to be helpful in keeping her symptoms in remission, although she held out hope that one day she wouldn't need them. Following the retirement of her previous psychiatrist, she had been consulting with me for about a year while continuing to see her long-term psychotherapist. Although free of significant depression, she often felt discouraged about herself and her prospects. Her experience of consistent equanimity over the past several years was only just beginning to give her a fresh sense of who she might be and what might be possible for her life.

In her meeting with me the week before I wrote this chapter, Anne, a plump, petite woman, said she was tired, but I also noticed that her usually careworn face had a bit of a glow. Her tiredness stemmed from a pleasing source: she had, after living for twenty-seven years in the same rental apartment, bought a house, and had moved in the previous week. In sitting with her, I was aware that she was dog-tired, but that also, under the surface, she felt incipient joy and perhaps even pride. Those were unprecedented emotions in our meetings, and I gently made space for them and invited them forward, through my joining in Anne's happiness and lingering in the telling of her experience of moving in. Here is a reconstruction of our conversation, as I captured it right after our meeting from my notes:

S: Congratulations, Anne! Wow.

ANNE: Thank you.

S: So now of course you're exhausted.

ANNE: Yes, I sure am.

S: What a big step, to buy your own house.

ANNE: Yes, as soon as I saw that house, I knew that it was my house.

S: Wow, you knew it was your house? How did you know?

ANNE: I don't know exactly. I just knew.

S: What a good feeling that must have been. What kind of a house is it?

ANNE: It's a ranch.

S: So it's all one level.

ANNE: Yes, which is nice because my apartment was on the second floor. Lots of up and down the stairs, especially moving.

S: Does it have a yard?

ANNE: Yes, a nice one, but bigger than I like, there will be a lot of mowing and raking.

S: And is there a patio?

ANNE: A screened breezeway, where I can sit.

S: Nice. Is it in the country or in town?

ANNE: It's near Cold Spring, so it's kind of in the country. It's weird that it's so quiet.

S: It's weird and new for it to be so quiet, but do you think you will like it?

ANNE: Yes. It's in a nice little neighborhood. In fact, a few days after I moved in, there was a knock on the door and there was a little boy with a plate of warm muffins. His mother was holding a vase of flowers and they said, "We'd like to welcome you to the neighborhood."

S: How was that for you?

ANNE: It was great. I asked the boy what grade he was in. "Kindergarten." I said, "So do the kids in this neighborhood go trick or treating?" And he said, "Oh yes!" "So do you think I should I get some candy?" "Oh yes!"

We laughed together. Anne was radiant. Through the course of this conversation, joy rose in her like the sun. My making space for and joining with Anne in her happiness offered the opportunity to take a step in developing the narrative of her life that included that happiness and promoted a positive sense of her own identity.

S: I'm wondering if moving to this new house gives you a new sense of yourself?

ANNE: Yes. Well, now I'm pretty exhausted from the move, but once I settle in I can tell I will feel excited about living there.

S: Now you are still tired, but you know you will be excited about living there. I can see that excitement in you. You seem really happy. I'm so glad for you! And that excitement and happiness in moving to your own house, I'm wondering if that has made a difference in your sense of who you are?

ANNE: Sometimes it feels like I haven't done anything with my life. I never married, I don't have children, but with the house I feel like I have done something with my life.

S: Buying this house—your house—and moving in gives you a sense that you have really done something with your life.

ANNE: Yes. (with quiet pride.) Yes, I have done something with my life.

What a tender and yet powerful new story Anne has created for herself in this brief conversation: *I have done something with my life.* My unabashed celebrating with Anne the momentousness of her buying and moving into her own house let her know that I would be able to hear exactly how meaningful it was to her. Together, we discovered that in addition to feeling tired, she felt excited and happy, and we coauthored a new story of pride and identity. My hearing and sharing in that story invigorated and solidified it as a source of strength for Anne. My empathic attunement made space for her to tell an emotionally moving story in a way that furthered her well-being.

## COLLABORATION, TRANSPARENCY AND CULTURAL ATTUNEMENT

Emotional attunement paves the way for a healing therapeutic alliance in which our patients feel deeply respected. In narrative psychiatry, we are seeking to help our patients live more as they prefer, in accordance with what they care most about, rather than imposing our personal, professional, or cultural view of well-being on them. While empathy is a hallmark of every therapeutic tradition, the empathy that is uniquely characteristic of narrative psychiatry arises from the deep respect that patients feel in having their own values and perspectives honored, in combination with the sense of connection they feel in being held in emotional attunement. Many things can contribute to creating respectful, empathic treatment relationships, including collaboration, transparency, and cultural attunement.

Collaboration means we work with our patients side by side as partners to determine the nature of the problems they are facing, and to consider what treatment options might be helpful. As narrative psychotherapists and psychiatrists, we seek to be in a consultative role with the patient, rather than an authoritative one. This "decentered but influential"[3] stance of narrative practice distinguishes it from treatment-as-usual. There is no one-size-fits-all treatment in narrative psychiatry, because we can't know in advance what is most important to our patients as they seek well-being. Rather, patients are honored as the authors of their lives and their identities, and our role is to be of service in helping our patients be able to live more as they uniquely prefer. While we may be experts about psychiatric and psychotherapeutic resources, our patients are the experts on their lives.

Transparency means that we are open with our patients about what we are doing in their treatment and why. Doing so conveys respect and promotes trust. Transparency serves to further empower our patients in

### Key Ideas about Therapeutic Relationships in Narrative Psychiatry

The meanings we give our experiences and feelings—the stories that make us who we are—arise in relationships.

Telling an emotionally moving story in a way that is healing requires an emotionally attuned listener.

Collaboration means working side by side with our patients as partners to determine the nature of the problems they are facing and to consider treatment options.

In narrative psychiatry, we seek a "decentered but influential"[4] stance in which we are in a consultative role with the patient, rather than an authoritative one.

Developing cultural attunement with our patients through understanding the wider contexts in which they and we are living promotes a healing therapeutic alliance.

Addressing the impact on patients' lives of racial, cultural, sexual, gender, and other identities and narratives, with sensitivity to issues of privilege and marginalization, builds trust and supports understanding.

Being transparent with our patients about what we are doing in their treatment and why conveys respect and promotes trust.

Empowering patients as partners in the treatment process promotes recovery because patients are better able to clarify and voice what they personally value and need.

the treatment relationship. There is an inherent power differential in doctor-patient relationships that transparency helps to mitigate. It promotes recovery when our patients have more power in treatment because they are better able to clarify and voice what they personally value and need.

Developing a healing therapeutic alliance with our patients also means understanding the wider contexts in which they—and we—are living. We can think of this as cultural attunement. We humans are cultural creatures. What we do and what we think, how we play and work and love, is shaped by the cultures in which we live. Our cultural contexts not only constrain and support us; they influence our experience of ourselves—our identities and how we feel. Narrative psychiatry invites us to bring the insights of narrative analysis to understand the social and cultural contexts in which we and our patients live. The customs and norms of our cultures and subcultures evolve in concert with cultural narratives about them. Illuminating cultural discourses allows us to better understand the ways in which they are affecting our patients' and our lives.

Why is awareness of cultural narratives important in connecting with our patients? First, because cultural discourses have an intimate effect on who we are as doctors and therapists and what we value. To understand and connect with our patients, especially across differences, we need to understand our own cultural identities and the cultural narratives that are influencing us, including those relating to concepts of illness and health. We need to know where we are coming from. Second, cultural discourses have an intimate effect on our patients' lives and identities. We cannot understand our patients if we do not understand the contexts in which they are living. They want to know that we get it. Third, addressing the impact on our patients' lives of racial, cultural, sexual, gender, and other identities, with sensitivity to issues of privilege and oppression, makes these cultural narratives explicit in the treatment relationship. Not only does this provide opportunities to interrogate and renegotiate these narratives; it helps to build trust, especially across cultural differences. Our patients want to know that we are allies.

Vanessa Jones was referred to me urgently last January by her psychotherapist. Vanessa had come to the university to obtain her PhD in social work with an emphasis on social justice. She had relocated from San Francisco where she had had a supportive community of friends and a job that she valued. Her therapist let me know that Vanessa was feeling isolated, stressed, and depressed; couldn't fall asleep for hours; and was having suicidal thoughts. She had had depression in the past that had been treated with citalopram. Her therapist wondered if medicine might be helpful now.

Vanessa, a petite, attractive woman with a clear, golden-brown complexion and smooth, dark hair pulled neatly back in a clip, entered my office and sat upright on the edge of my couch. Her shoulders were hunched and she spoke warily about her current stresses. Yes, she was depressed, but no, she did not want antidepressants, just something to help her sleep. I felt her sadness and worry and pride. I was aware that she was a woman of color, that I was white and that we were meeting in the context of a white-dominated university in which she said she felt isolated. To begin to bring cultural issues into our conversation, I asked her what her ethnic background was. She replied that her father was African American and her mother was Filipino.

"And how are things for you culturally here at UMass?" I asked. My hope with this question was to convey that I assumed that culture was relevant to her experience, that her experience was hers alone to define, and that I could hear whatever she might have to say, including any experiences of racism. Vanessa hesitantly replied that it was hard being a woman of color in a new, predominantly white environment when she didn't yet have a community of people of color who could support her. She had had a strong community back in San Francisco that she really missed, and she was wondering if she had made a mistake in coming to graduate school so far away. As we spoke about these cultural issues Vanessa looked at me discerningly.

"You present as white, so…." she said. I understood the subtext to be, *Since you enjoy white privilege, I don't know how much of my experience as a woman of color you can understand.* This was an important moment where transparency and cultural awareness could foster connection and, I hoped, a healing therapeutic alliance. I responded by saying that I was from a European American background, and that I wondered if she was worried that because I was white, I wouldn't be able to understand her experience as a woman of color. This reflection further strengthened the bridge across our differences that we were building together. As we continued to speak about issues of race and culture and gender, Vanessa could hear that I knew something about the operations of racism and how debilitating it was to experience racist micro-aggressions on a daily basis, especially without a community of support. In speaking of these things together, we developed greater ease and trust, and I could see Vanessa begin to relax with me a bit. We were developing cultural attunement.

I was transparent with her about my concern about the extent of the depression she was experiencing, as it included thoughts of suicide, but Vanessa was clear that she was not intending to harm herself and that she didn't want anti-depressant medications. She just wanted something to help her sleep. I respected her preferences and prescribed a low dose of trazodone as a sleep aid and scheduled an appointment to see her again in ten days.

At our next appointment, Vanessa was more comfortable with me. She noted that she was feeling better after spending time with friends in Boston. She reported that the trazodone was helping her sleep through the night, but she continued to have low mood, decreased interest in things, and a sense of isolation, with some fleeting suicidal thoughts that were not urgent. We spoke about her experiences as a graduate student. She noted that she felt compelled to speak up about injustice in her classes, but felt there was a high cost for doing so. We discussed the meaning of using antidepressants in contexts in which social injustice was contributing to feelings of depression, putting our heads together to examine cultural narratives about the nature of suffering, wellness, privilege, and oppression. Together we weighed the pros and cons of resuming citalopram. Vanessa concluded that her goal of promoting social justice by getting her PhD could be best served by treating her symptoms of depression with weekly psychotherapy with her therapist, and possibly by taking an antidepressant. She took a prescription for citalopram.

At our next appointment three weeks later, Vanessa reported that she had been taking steps to support her well-being, including weekly psychotherapy, seeing new friends, staying connected with close friends from San Francisco, mindfulness practices, and exercise, but she continued to experience symptoms of depression that interfered with her ability to complete her coursework, which included suicidal thoughts. She had not filled the prescription, saying it seemed like a sign of weakness to resort to using antidepressants. I was aware at this moment of the range of narratives in circulation about the nature of depression and the use of medicine to treat it, as well as the values that Vanessa herself held and the narratives she favored, such as those espousing the value of social justice for those with less privilege. I wondered if her narrative that antidepressants were a sign of weakness reflected the imposition on her of a dominant cultural story that ran counter to her values, or if it was, indeed, a reflection of her own values.

Opening up cultural narratives to scrutiny reveals the values and ideas on which they are based, which lets our patients decide how well those narratives fit their own values. Similarly to how we exposed the operations of cultural discourses that promoted racism, Vanessa and I could deconstruct discourses about mental health symptoms. In doing so, I was aware that I needed to take great care not to impose my own values on her; namely, that taking antidepressants was *not* a sign of weakness. At the same time, a thorough look at the cultural narratives about psychotropic medicines could help Vanessa further clarify her perspectives.

Together we noted that cultural narratives that made disparaging identity claims about using medicine to treat symptoms of depression were perhaps even more predominant in African American and Filipino cultures than in European American ones. We contrasted the narratives about using antidepressants with narratives about using anti-asthma medicines, which made no negative claims about the character of those who used an inhaler when it was hard to breathe. We noted the similarities between asthma and depression, both of which can be exacerbated by environmental factors and stress. Ultimately, we compared the underlying values of the narrative that said it was a sign of weakness to use an antidepressant with Vanessa's own values, which were that it actually took strength of character to persist in seeking to overcome depression. She realized that she felt sad that her depression had recurred to the extent that antidepressant medicines were being considered, and she was reluctant to give up hope that she might be able to recover without them. She would continue to weigh the pros and cons of starting citalopram, and I supported her choice.

Three weeks later, Vanessa reported that she was feeling much better. In addition to all her other efforts to recover, she had started the citalopram and believed that it was helpful.

As the months went on, Vanessa continued to support her well-being in many ways. She clarified her vision for promoting social justice as a scholar of social work and felt a sense of "intrinsic motivation" in pursuing that goal. She succeeded in creating a supportive community of people of color for herself locally, her own "gang of friends." She noted that in the larger university it was continuously taxing to feel a sense of cultural alienation, but with her gang she felt she could be her "full self." When I asked her if there were any other places in her life where she felt she could be her full self, she said, "Yes, with my therapist, and here, with you."

## VANESSA'S REFLECTIONS

Soon after I finished writing this chapter, I sent it to Vanessa to read for accuracy and I invited her to write a reflection. In the e-mail she sent to me she said, "I was able to read the book chapter you sent me and I feel completely comfortable with the representation of our sessions together."

Here is the reflection she wrote:

> In my experience as a woman of color, I personally take many things into consideration before I seek counseling. Initially, I feel burdened by the cultural stigma given my Black and Asian background that traditionally demands that one should be stoic in the face of adversity and I should only share my problems with family and close friends. I worry I will be perceived as weak for

seeking professional help from someone who has no connection to my personal life and who is often White. It has been my experience that the internal negotiation about whether to seek treatment is a mentally and emotionally draining process that does not end once I have made the decision to get counseling. I then worry about how the actual counseling experience will be if my therapist/doctor is White. Will they understand the constant presence and operation of privilege and oppression in my life? Will they relate to me if our cultural, educational and class backgrounds are different and what kind of bias and discrimination should I be prepared for? To what extent will I encounter a White doctor who may believe in colorblindness, denies present day racism, sexism, etc., has stereotypical assumptions, believes in the myth of meritocracy, or worse, provides me culturally insensitive treatment?

When I first met with Dr. Hamkins, I was in an incredibly vulnerable state and looking back now, I would have been more wounded if not for the cultural competency she displayed. She built rapport with me by showing she understood that cultural identifiers such as race, sex and class are embedded in my lived reality as a person who identifies as a woman of color. She allowed me to be the expert of my own narrative; her office was a safe place where I did not have to worry about the social construction of normativity, I could discuss openly and honestly my struggles, including those that are due to social conditions.

A doctor who is comfortable with having difficult conversations, especially around race, was significant in our cross-racial collaboration to navigate my treatment. It honored my experience as a person of color and how my own cultural narrative influences my sense of self and my resiliency. I am happy to share that the understanding patient/doctor relationship we built is part of my growing self-awareness, the satisfaction in my treatment, and my ability to advocate for myself.

## Notes

1. Daniel Siegel, *The Mindful Therapist: A Clinician's Guide to Mindsight and Neural Integration* (New York: W. W. Norton, 2010), 36.
2. Emotional attunement has always been an implicit value and practice of narrative psychiatry and narrative therapy, although it has rarely been explicitly addressed as such. More detail and evidence about the developmental and healing aspects of emotional attunement and resonance can be found in Siegel, *The Mindful Therapist,* 1–87.
3. White, *Maps,* 39.
4. Ibid., 39.

# CHAPTER THREE

# Starting with Stories of Success

## The Initial Psychiatric Consultation

If compassionate connection is the heart of narrative psychiatry, then eliciting healing stories is its soul. In narrative psychiatry, we begin seeking stories of strength and meaning from the very first appointment. As we listen to the story a patient brings to us, we also listen for the untold stories implicit in their narrative that may support their well-being. Fleshing out these stories, making them alive with detail, vivid with language and compelling with plot, strengthens them and gives them purchase to eclipse a disempowering, problem-dominated story.

What we can know about a patient depends on what we are listening for. The openings for story development that we hear and the questions we ask in the first appointment lead to the cocreation of the narrative of the patient's life that informs our understanding of the problem and our treatment options. By eliciting narratives that lead to a more nuanced, colorful, and balanced portrait of the patient and a more contextualized view of the problem, we can understand the nature of the problem and the patient with more depth, clarity and subtlety.

## NARRATIVE APPROACHES TO INITIAL PSYCHIATRIC CONSULTATIONS: AMANDA'S STORY

What might this look like in practice?

Tall and thin with a short spiky haircut, and carrying a canvas messenger bag, Amanda Riley spoke earnestly when she first came in to see me for treatment of depression. A sophomore in college, she was mired in a story of how she was making bad decisions and wasn't living her life right. Amanda had been referred to me by a psychotherapist at the college counseling service where I consulted due to concerns about panic attacks and depressed mood. The hope was that I would be able to help Amanda clarify the nature of the problem and determine if medication might be helpful, a typical workaday situation for many psychiatrists in today's world.

So how would a narrative psychiatrist approach his or her first meeting with Amanda?

At the start of my initial conversation with Amanda, I asked her what year of school she was in and what she was studying. She told me she was a sophomore in college, majoring in Chinese and art. At this point in the interview I might have chosen to get a much fuller history of what has drawn Amanda to Chinese and art, to find and bring more fully into the light of day stories about her values and strengths, but I could tell from her demeanor that she was eager to talk about what was bothering her, so that was where I began.

I try to discern from the way patients respond to my initial questions whether they would prefer to speak first about who they are and what they care about, or about the problem that has led them to consult with me. Following the patient's preference facilitates empathic attunement and fosters a collaborative therapeutic relationship, and this was my intention with Amanda. Although it is possible to ask directly about these preferences, I am sensitive to the power relations at play when someone consults with a psychiatrist. The person consulting is aware that discourses of medicine and psychiatry often privilege the perspectives of psychiatrists over the perspectives of people who consult with psychiatrists. They may be concerned that they will have identity conclusions and treatments imposed on them. The power of the discourses that lead to this sort of imposition is such that it is generally not helpful to ask someone at the beginning of their first meeting with me about their preferences regarding which questions I ask them. They may experience a question about their preferences as some kind of test or trick, or they may be confused. The result is that they feel even more disempowered than if I hadn't asked their preference. My decision at this point about what direction to go in—construction or deconstruction, so to speak—is based on my sense of their comfort and interest in the questions I ask about their life and what they care about.

So in Amanda's case, I asked her about the problem early in the interview.[1]

S:  What brings you in to see me?

AMANDA: I've been depressed, and I think I need medication.

S:  What has the depression been like?

AMANDA: I feel like I just want to get out of my skin. I've been isolating myself in my room and dwelling on my problems. I'm unsure of myself and that makes me feel even more down on myself. Nothing I'm doing to try to feel better is working. I'm doing a bad job on my schoolwork, and I don't even know what I want to be studying for. I feel scared about what's coming up next in my life, like I should be doing a better job of knowing what I want.… I feel like I'm arbitrarily redefining things.… Overall, I feel like I am making bad decisions about my life and not living my life right.

You can hear the story that Amanda told about the meaning of what she was experiencing. She faced challenges in not yet knowing what she wanted to study in college and not doing as well as she wanted academically, and she understood those challenges according to the plot line, "I am making bad decisions and not living my life right." My thought was that this theme might be contributing to her suffering, and I anticipated finding openings for developing new narratives after I have heard a full account of her concerns.

In this conversation, you can also hear that the first time the problem is mentioned, I offered an externalized description of it. By *externalized* I mean a description of the problem as separate from the person's identity[2]. When I paraphrased her statement "I've been depressed" with my phrase "the depression," Amanda responded by offering a rich and meaningful description of her experience. Most people welcome an externalized description of what was a negative identity conclusion. They experience relief in changing the description of the problem from an adjective describing them to a noun affecting them.

In my conversation with Amanda, I proceeded to develop the history of the problem's influence on her, in an externalized way. From the many different people who have told me about the ways that depression has been disruptive in their lives and from my studies in psychiatry, I know that at times depression can cause a whole group of negative effects. My next questions were designed to understand if Amanda's depression was causing some of these problems.

S: Is the depression interfering with your concentration?

AMANDA: Yes! I can't concentrate at all and it's hard to get my work done.

S: Has the depression influenced your sleep?

AMANDA: I'm sleeping all the time, and it's still hard getting up in the morning.

S: Does the depression bring thoughts that life is not worth living?

AMANDA: Once in a while I do get thoughts of taking my life, but I know I would never do that.

S: When did the depression first appear?

AMANDA: Since February, about two months ago.

You can hear multiple examples of externalization in these questions. The low-key, redundant description of her problem in an externalized way conveyed to Amanda she is not the depression, that the depression is unwanted, and that she is not to blame for the effects of the depression. This offers an alternative to the self-blaming narrative

Amanda came in with. Externalization works against negative identity conclusions and tangibly changes the person's experience of the problem. Gathering information this way feels better to patients. It's therapeutic. Explaining or pointing to the process of externalization is not necessary for people to benefit from it. They simply experience the difference. However, at times making the process of externalization more overt can be helpful in creating new stories that support a person's priorities and preferences. (I'll say more about externalizing and unpacking problems in chapter 4.)

Next in my conversation with Amanda, I developed the history of her resistance to the problem, as fully, or more fully, than the history of the problem's influence on her. Everyone who consults with a psychiatrist or psychotherapist has been attempting to resist their problems. My goal was to open space to illuminate all the ways in which someone has been and might be successful in limiting the influence of the problem in their life.[3]

S: When do you feel the best nowadays?
AMANDA: When I'm doing art.

I was a little surprised by her answer. From what I knew about depression, it tends to make it difficult if not impossible to engage in any self-motivated creativity, let alone to feel best doing so. Prior to working narratively, my questions might have ended here, and I might have simply encouraged Amanda to "do more art." But in narrative work, the goal is first to notice and then to develop the story of this "unique outcome."[4] It's an opening for developing an entirely new narrative. A unique outcome is an experience or idea, no matter how small, that stands apart from the problem or the problem's usual effects. It is a bit of evidence of the person's success in living as they prefer despite the problem.

On its own, one unique experience isn't a story, and it doesn't have much power to offer new meaning to a person's experience. But when it is connected with other similar events according to a theme, a new narrative emerges. As narrative psychiatrists, we seek out the kernel of a story that explains a unique outcome, and then we generate compelling tellings of this story. That is, we seek out the same things that make for good literature: ravishing detail, memorable language, singular characters, dramatic plot lines.

The story of how someone is succeeding in resisting her problems is one we cannot know ahead of time. Only the person resisting knows exactly how she is doing it. This is one of many reasons why our work in narrative psychiatry must be collaborative.

S:  It's unexpected to me that you are able to enjoy making art despite the depression. How are you able to do this?

AMANDA:  I wasn't always able to enjoy making art, but I learned to say to myself: I'm learning a skill. It may not be perfect. This is a process. I'm doing this because I enjoy it. I don't have to have so many expectations of what it has to be like.

S:  Wait, let me be sure I can get all this down! (writing furiously) *I'm learning a skill. It may not be perfect. This is a process. I'm doing this because I enjoy it. I don't have to have so many expectations…*

AMANDA:  So many expectations of what the art has to be like. I learned to take a break when I got frustrated. I used to destroy art I made that I didn't like, but I disciplined myself to tolerate my less successful work. I learned to say to myself, *I have to make bad art on the way to making good art. This is necessary to become an artist.*

S:  (Still writing.) You learned to say, *I have to make bad art on the way to making good art. This is necessary to become an artist.*

As Amanda offered the story of how she has learned to be able to enjoy making art even in the face of depression, I wrote down and repeated out loud all the things she said to further strengthen her knowledge through my saying them and her hearing them.

When I had a detailed, lively, and full account of the development of her skill in resisting negative appraisal of her art and in promoting her artistic self-development, then I sought to develop this alternative story into other areas of her life and across time. In doing so, we were continuing to cocreate a narrative of Amanda's life that would offer her a way of understanding and telling the story of her current dilemma that fits with identity conclusions that she found invigorating. In seeking to generate a rich alternative tapestry, there are always many different threads of the story that may be taken up and more vividly developed. In this conversation, for example, I could have chosen to thicken the story of Amanda's connection to art, or to elicit the particulars of how she learned to tolerate "bad art." Here is what I did do:

S:  I'm wondering if this same philosophy of looking at making art as a process could also be applied to your life in general. I'm wondering whether or not figuring out what you want to do with your life is something of an art, and if you can say some of the same things, such as: "I'm learning a skill" and "This is a process."

AMANDA:  (Her face lights up.) Yes! I never thought of it that way!

We went on to discuss ways in which figuring out her life may involve making decisions, such as about her major, her friendships, and her priorities, and about how she was trying to find a balance between allowing for openness without losing control or becoming apathetic. We discussed her sources of inspiration in the process of living her life.

At the conclusion of our fifty-minute conversation, Amanda reported feeling more relaxed and optimistic, feeling that she knew how to steer her life in the directions in which she wishes it to go while being open to new possibilities. She said she was feeling much better, and was no longer interested in antidepressant medications.

I offered to send her a synopsis of our conversation, which she welcomed, as a way to further flesh out and support her new story about herself. It was a help to me that I had the resources to dictate this letter and have it typed for me, and that it served as part of the medical record documentation of our meeting.

Dear Amanda,

I am writing to summarize some of the points of our conversation to provide documentation to you of some of the things that you have been doing that have been useful in helping yourself to successfully live your life.

You noted that the days you feel best are the days you go into the art studio and spend time making art. You have been able to continue to make art despite depression because of being able to say the following things to yourself:

- I'm learning a skill.

- It may not be perfect.

- This is a process.

- I'm doing this because I enjoy it.

- I don't have to have so many expectations of what it has to be like.

In addition, you are able to take a break when you become frustrated with yourself, and also you are able to resist doing things that are destructive to your work or to yourself. Furthermore, you are able to say to yourself: "I have to do this work to move toward a goal."

You are considering whether the same philosophy of looking at art as a process might also be applied to living your life in general. You are considering whether or not thinking that figuring out what you want to do with your life is something of an art, and that saying to yourself some of the same things such as: "I'm learning a skill" and "This is a process" may be useful in allowing you to relax and let other things surface.

You have described several sources of inspiration to you currently, including: art, plays, women you admire, and professors. In particular, you note that people who are able to work with what they have and make the most of it are especially inspiring and you are considering speaking to some people and interviewing them about how they are able to do this. Other sources of inspiration include: hard physical labor, being outdoors, making friends, and spending time with people.

You mentioned that you thought being able to read a document such as this might be useful to you in creating more space in your life for relaxation and optimism, and might help you to direct your life in directions you wish while being open to new possibilities.

This letter itself can be considered a work in progress. Please feel free to bring this to our next meeting and also to make any corrections that seem appropriate to you so that this document can be most accurate and helpful.

I look forward to speaking with you at our next conversation.

Sincerely,
SuEllen Hamkins, MD
College Psychiatrist

---

Amanda continued in brief psychotherapy with the therapist who had referred her to me, and her depression resolved without medications. One year later, Amanda consulted with me again. She reported that our conversation the previous year had been very helpful, and that her depression had faded as she became more active and made new friends. She presented now with some specific relationship concerns she wished to speak about in individual therapy, and met with a psychotherapist for several sessions. One year after that, she engaged in a psychotherapy group with the intention of enhancing her abilities to express her feelings in intimate relationships.

This interview illustrates how empathically connecting with the patient, externalizing the problem, and gathering a full, richly detailed, emotionally meaningful history of resistance to the problem in an initial psychiatric consultation is therapeutic. In narrative psychiatry, the initial psychiatric consultation is a collaborative conversation in which a new story of meaning and identity can emerge.

## DEVELOPING A HISTORY OF RESISTANCE TO THE PROBLEM

There are many kinds of questions that can be asked to develop a history of resistance to a problem in the context of an initial psychiatric consultation. I like how the phrase "history of resistance to the problem" stands in contrast to "history of the problem," commonly seen as a heading in psychiatric or psychological reports. "History of resistance to the problem" is another way of saying "counterplot" or "alternative storyline." Some of my favorite questions to start developing a history of resistance to the problem include *When do you feel best nowadays?* and *What helped you get through that difficult time?* These and other questions listed in the box "Sample Questions to Develop a History of Resistance to the Problem" can be an entry point for a rich conversation in which a person can discover how they have been successful in resisting their problems and living according to their most precious values.

---

**Sample Questions to Develop a History of Resistance to the Problem**

When do you feel the best nowadays?

What helped you get through that difficult time?

Are there times that the problem doesn't get to you?

Are there values that you have been able to stay true to despite feeling down?

Are there times you were able to resist the urges to cut? How did you do it?

What have you been doing to try to limit the effects of worrying?

Are there things you are doing to try to keep the voices in the background?

Are there actions you have taken to help with concentration?

---

No matter how severe or intractable a problem is, the person facing it is always trying to resist it. The story of their efforts and successes in resistance is often invisible both to them and to others. It is vital in psychiatric settings to elicit this alternative story. The story of resistance to the problem is the compass and map that leads out of the landscape dominated by the problem, and it directs our patients to the provisions and companions needed to help forge a new, more satisfying path. Developing in our first contact the narrative of a patient's efforts and successes in resisting the problem fosters a strengths-based foundation for treatment that supports recovery.

In narrative psychiatry, rather than privileging only stories of loss, suffering, conflict, neglect, or abuse in someone's life, I also search for stories of joy, connection, intimacy, consistency, and success, for these are the wealth of the people who consult with us. Instead of privileging a story of failure, we coauthor a story of successes in overcoming problems, no matter how small those successes may be.

Seeking out descriptions of family history that describe close and supportive relationships between family members stands in contrast to only seeking descriptions that highlight painful aspects of family life. I often ask, "Who are you closest to in your family?" and "What does your partner [or mother or friend] especially love or appreciate about you?"

The change in focus to success in resisting a problem is especially helpful in dealing with problems that can be serious and long-standing, such as self-injury. For example, we can find an externalized description of the problem near to the experience, such as "the urge to cut," and then look for successful resistance. We can ask:

- Has there been a time when you had an urge to cut and you didn't?
- How did you resist?

We seek a detailed description of the person's experiences, actions, feelings, and thoughts as she engaged in this act of resistance. Each aspect of her resistance is evidence of her skill and commitment in overcoming the urge to cut. For example, she may have the skill of talking herself out of cutting (*You can get through this without cutting*), skills of self-soothing (taking a bath, going for a walk, listening to music), skills of reminding herself of her commitment to refrain from self-harm, skills of connecting with loved ones, and so on.

Each skill in resisting has a history that may be developed:

- Have you ever done that before? When was the first time?

- Did you learn to comfort yourself in that way on your own, or did someone help you learn that?

Each action of resistance in the present and past has meanings, values, and commitments connected with it that can be highlighted and strengthened:

- Does your desire not to worry your family about your safety reflect a value you hold?

- Does your plan to eliminate cutting from your life reflect commitments you have for your life?

It's not uncommon for someone to answer the question, *How did you manage to resist?* with the response, *I don't know.* Our work is clear: find out how. The person has skills he doesn't know he possesses.

## QUESTIONS THAT GENERATE EXPERIENCE AND GATHER INFORMATION

In addition to holding ourselves responsible for asking questions that are therapeutic, as psychiatrists and clinicians we also hold ourselves responsible for understanding the nature of a problem troubling someone. If there are biological aspects to the problem, psychiatrists are responsible for understanding how they are likely to play out over time and how they are likely to respond to various resources the person may choose to draw upon, including medicines. Fully understanding the nature of a problem means gathering information about it.

To fulfill our responsibility to gather information for understanding a problem *and* our responsibility to ask questions that generate therapeutic experiences, we need to gather information in ways that attend to the effects of the gathering. Luckily, this is easy to do. In fact, questions that gather information provide rich opportunities for more fully developing a preferred storyline.

For example, understanding the nature of a problem includes knowing when it first occurred and how it evolved over time. Revitalizing identity conclusions can be supported and information can be gathered by asking questions such as the following:

- Have you ever gotten over depression before?
- When was that?
- How did you do it?

The question *How did you do it?* is a gateway to coauthoring new narratives, such as that described in Amanda's case. But in addition to supporting identity conclusions that honor a person's preferences, skills, and knowledge, focusing on how someone overcame a problem in the past also instructs the psychiatrist in the particular resources that this person found helpful in doing so.

Likewise, understanding the nature of a problem that may have a biological component includes understanding whether biological family members share the problem, because there is a genetic component to many psychiatric problems. For example, if someone has identified their problem as a serious depression, it is helpful to know if other biological family members have had mood problems, and if so, what kind. Therefore, in addition to understanding the resources of love and support that person may have in their family, the narrative psychiatrist is also gathering information about whether family members have also faced similar problems as the consulting person and how family members are resisting those problems. Describing problems in an externalized way mitigates blame and a sense of failure. In this way, a family history is developed that simultaneously attends to gathering information and generating experience. The kinds of questions that can be asked include the following:

- Is anyone else in your family being tormented by depression?
- In what ways do you see them resisting the depression?
- How many times did your mother succeed in regaining her equilibrium after a manic episode? How did she do it?

**Sample Questions to Develop a Positive Family History**

Who in your family are you closest to?

What do they love or admire about you?

Is that an indication of what your family gives value to?

What would you say are some of the things your family cares most about?

Is there anyone else in your family who has worked to overcome depression? What have they done to resist its influence in their life?

Is anyone in your family dealing with the challenge of bipolar disorder? What has their strategy been to limit its effects?

Have any family members had a problem with alcohol or drugs? Have they in any way tried to minimize its negative effects on the family? What did they do?

Every piece of information that is relevant to understanding and resisting a problem can be gathered in a way that is therapeutic.

## THERAPEUTIC DOCUMENTATION

The stories of strength and meaning that we develop with our patients can be reflected in our medical records. Records we keep about our patients are, of course, narratives about their lives. What we say in those narratives guides our understanding of our patients and our therapeutic practices, as well as the understanding and practices of other clinicians who read them. Narratives that focus predominantly on problems and deficits paint a negative and impoverished portrait of our patients and obscure the strengths, resources, and intentions that are the foundation of recovery—yet such problem-dominated narratives typify psychiatric records today. We can easily change that.

Creating medical records that offer balanced narratives of our patients' strengths and values as well as their problems is very straightforward, whether we are working with existing psychiatry-as-usual documentation standards or creating our own. While the traditional mental health record requires us to tell the story of our patients' problems, organized in sections such as Chief Complaint, History of Present Illness, Psychiatric History, Medical History, Family History, and Clinical Impression, it is not difficult to include in these same sections the story of our patients' hopes for consultation and vision of well-being, their current successes in resisting their problems and the history of those successes, their practices that promote their physical health, their families' strengths and values, and a summary of their resiliencies and resources. When I worked at a community mental health center with traditional documentation expectations, this is what I did. (For an example, see Maeli's story in the Introduction.)

Narrative-psychiatry-informed documentation invites us to tell an even more robust story of strength and meaning. In my private practice, I created a template that foregrounded rich descriptions of my patients' intentions, successes, and resources while clearly describing the problems they were facing. At times, I would use letters as documentation, such as the one I wrote to Amanda. Recently, at The Center for Counseling & Psychological Health at the University of Massachusetts–Amherst, drawing inspiration from the work of Bill Madsen,[5] colleagues[6] and I collaborated in creating strengths-based electronic medical record forms that elicit narratives about patients' passions and interests, their goals for treatment, the nature of their problems and their successes in resisting them, areas of life that are going well, and the strengths and vulnerabilities of their families and what family members value about them, and that include a summary that invites mention of patients' strengths, skills, resiliencies, supports, and cultural values as well as problems, obstacles, and psychiatric diagnoses. My overall intention is to create records that are thorough, point the way toward recovery, and would be therapeutic if patients read them.

Documentation of an initial consultation or a referral to another clinician can begin with an introduction to the person, not the problem. In this, I am guided by practices of introduction that are respectful and honoring—that is, practices one might use when introducing esteemed

### A Template for Creating Strengths- and Values-Based Documentation of Initial Consultations

Introduction to the person without the problem:
  (Include passions, interests, values, skills, accomplishments, and
  sources of inspiration)
The person's goals for treatment and vision of well-being:
Chief concern:
History of the problem and efforts and successes in overcoming it:
Family history:
  (Include family values, skills, and resources; what family mem-
  bers admire about the person; and the problems that family
  members have faced and/or overcome)
Medical well-being and problems:
Observations/mental status:
Summary:
  (Include strengths, skills, relationships, supports, and values;
  successes in achieving their vision of well-being; and problems
  that are a focus of treatment)
Risk assessment:
  (Include risks for harm to self or others and protective factors)
Diagnoses, discussed with patient:
Collaborative treatment plan:

colleagues or friends. When we receive referrals from colleagues, we can invite them to offer us this kind of introduction to their patients. Just recently, when a psychotherapist called and began to tell me about all the problems of a patient he wanted me to see, I asked him, "What do you admire or appreciate about Ted?"

"What a great question!" he exclaimed. "No psychiatrist has ever asked me that before," and he proceeded to tell me about Ted's intelligence, fortitude, creativity, and commitment to social justice.

## SUMMARY OF NARRATIVE APPROACHES TO INITIAL PSYCHIATRIC CONSULTATIONS

To summarize, in narrative psychiatry the purpose of an initial consultation is to accomplish the following:

- Empathically connect with the patient.

- Learn about his or her cultural identity and experiences.

- Develop the story of what the patient values and hopes for.

- Come to a common understanding of the nature of the problem or problems that are constraining the patient, speaking about problems in an externalized way—that is, as separate from the patient's identity.

- Therapeutically gather information about the patient's family and medical history.

- Discover, strengthen, and extend into the future the story of the patient's skill and knowledge in resisting the problem and living as he or she prefers.

- Collaboratively identify personal and psychiatric resources that might contribute to his or her preferred ways of being.

The result is movement from a problem-dominated narrative to a strengths-based narrative that promotes a story of cherished values and preferred identity and supports actions that move a person closer to living as they prefer.

How does a narrative psychiatry initial consultation differ from psychiatric treatment-as-usual?

- The psychiatrist works collaboratively, in a side-by-side stance with the person who is seeking consultation.

- Problems are talked about in an externalized way.

- Full histories of resistance to the problem and of sources of inspiration and meaning are developed. As much or more time in the interview is spent on illuminating the person's effect on the problem as on the problem's effect on the person.

- Care is taken to elicit information in ways that the patient experiences as therapeutic.

- Medical records can offer balanced narratives of patients' strengths and values as well as their problems.

Since I began working narratively twelve years ago, there has been a change in how people feel when they leave my office after their initial consultation. My original training in psychiatry had taught me to focus in an initial consultation on finding out about the problem and everything that might have contributed to it, which basically elicited a description of every negative experience the person consulting with me had ever had, and he or she would leave weighed down with that burden. I also felt weighed down by that way of practicing. Now that I focus on the person's skills and preferences in resisting problems and in creating a life consistent with their cherished values, we both feel energized after our conversations. While psychiatry-as-usual asks only *Why are you having this problem?* narrative psychiatry also asks *Why are you not having it?*

## Notes

1. This dialogue is a reconstruction from my written notes taken during the conversation.
2. White, *Maps*, 9.
3. I draw inspiration in doing so from the "opening space questions" Jill Freedman and Gene Combs describe in their book, *Narrative Therapy*, 124.
4. White, *Maps*, 61.
5. William Madsen, *Collaborative Therapy with Multi-stressed Families*, 3rd ed. (New York: Guilford, 2007), and personal communication.
6. David Browne, Donna Kellogg, Jen LeFort, Eliza McArdle, Robyn Miller, and Harry Rockland-Miller.

# CHAPTER FOUR

# Externalizing and Unpacking the Problem

## *Understanding Symptoms and Suffering*

The person is not the problem, the problem is the problem.
—*Michael White*[1]

Seeing the problem as separate from the person is a stance that informs narrative psychiatry. This stance gives us firm footing in responding to our patients with respect and empathy and frees us to nimbly and creatively work with them to mitigate the unwanted effects of problems in their lives. We don't blame patients for their problems. Rather, we align with them side-by-side to look out at the problem together and see what can be done about it. What this means is seeing problems as separate from our patients' identities; that is, as outside of what they value and who they are striving to be. In doing so, we see both the problem and the person more clearly.

Externalizing the problem in this way is a therapeutic practice that is one of our most powerful narrative interventions. It shifts the psychological landscape in which we are working. Patients often experience their problems as all encompassing. By externalizing the problem, it becomes circumscribed and we can more easily unpack it: characterize it, determine its boundaries, discover how it is impinging on a person's life, expose the ways in which it operates, and discern what supports it and what weakens it. Separating the problem from the person makes it easier to see how patients are succeeding in living their lives in ways that they find satisfying and how they have freed themselves from the influence of the problem. We can more easily discover areas of the patient's life in which the problem is not operating or is powerless, and we can more readily discover strengths and resources that a patient can draw on to overcome the problem. Not seeing problems as integral to who patients are provides immediate relief from negative identity conclusions, which are often piled on top of other unwanted effects of problems. These discoveries are energizing, inspire hope, and point the way toward effective treatment.

The practice of externalization was developed by Michael White[2] as a way to objectify problems instead of objectifying people. Inspired by the work of Foucault,[3] who revealed how, in the modern world, people who experience mental health and other problems are subject to normative judgments that objectify them and assign them damaged identities, White wrote that understanding problems in an externalized way "makes it possible for people to experience an identity that is separate from the problem; the problem becomes the problem, not the person. In the context of externalizing conversations, the problem ceases to represent the 'truth' of about people's identities, and options for successful problem resolution suddenly become visible and accessible."[4] In addition, externalization enables us to situate the problem in its cultural and historical context; that is, to understand how cultural discourses contribute to the manifestations and effects of the problem.

In addition to offering us graceful ways to thoroughly understand the nature of problems, seeing them as separate from the person compels us to think in non-pathologizing ways about our patients. In working narratively, we resist the pull to see the patient's problem as an inevitable result of temperament, trauma, past experiences, present life circumstances, or character. It's not that trauma, the limitations of temperament, and difficult life experiences are not influential in people's lives—of course they are—but they do not *define* people's lives, and even more important, they do not point the way toward recovery. Focusing primarily on narratives of damage, limitations, and weaknesses strengthens those narratives and makes them more influential in our patients' lives—and more influential in our minds as therapists. An overemphasis on psychological theorizing about pathology can distract us from noticing the nuances of our patients' strengths and positive developments in their lives. Rather than focusing only or primarily on pathology, narrative psychiatry is interested in which aspects of our patients' characters or past experiences are *resources* for them.

As narrative psychiatrists, we are just as curious as other psychiatrists and psychotherapists about our patients' lives, characters, and temperaments. We listen with as much attention and nuance to their stories and body language, and we sift through their experiences of their lives with them with as much psychological perceptiveness and subtlety, but instead of primarily seeking the source of their problems, we are seeking the sources of their strengths. These are the resources that will help them move their lives in the directions that they prefer.

## EXTERNALIZING AND UNPACKING THE PROBLEM: WONJU'S STORY

When Wonju Lee first came to consult with me, she sat stiffly on the edge of my couch with her backpack at her feet and barely made eye contact. She had been referred to me by her psychotherapist for psychiatric consultation. A twenty-two-year-old Korean woman of average height and weight, Wonju had beautiful, clear skin and a constrained, somber expression on her round face. She was born in Korea, came to New York with her family for elementary school, then returned to Korea for middle and high school, and had come back to the United States for college, which she found culturally comfortable, although she missed her family. Just finishing her junior year, she was majoring in nursing, and her expression momentarily brightened when I asked her how she liked it: "I love it!" This was a beautiful opportunity to develop a story of success at the beginning of our first meeting, and I lingered here to thicken and enrich the story of what she loved and was good at. She said nursing really "hit home" with her, that it was interesting and had great opportunities for advancement, and that she was looking forward to a career as a nurse practitioner. At the university, she had a coveted full-time nursing research position for the summer.

She looked away and her expression again became stiff and sad when I asked her what her hopes were for our consultation. She said it was hard for her to speak of the problem that brought her in to see me, because she felt so embarrassed by it. In fact, she had delayed coming in for consultation for over a year, but now wanted to get help. She took a breath and said, "I've been trying to quit purging but it's not working." Given how hard it was for her to bring up this topic, I directed my attention first to understanding the problem and filed the "I've been trying to quit" part of her statement for later exploration. In this I was paying attention to my emotional attunement with Wonju.

In coming to understand the nature of the problem that is troubling someone, our task is to develop a detailed description of the problem that is both externalized and experience near. That is, we want to know how the person experiences the problem impinging on his or her life. Getting the details circumscribes the problem and lays it bare for scrutiny. With Wonju, I gently asked, "How is purging currently present in your life?" You can hear the externalization implicit in this phrasing. She noted that the purging had been occurring once or twice every day for over a year. Sometimes she was drawn into overeating to the point of pain or until she physically couldn't eat anymore, then she would purge by vomiting. She would try to eat a healthy amount, but she noted that she would still purge even if she hadn't overeaten. Currently, sessions of overeating and vomiting usually happened at night when she was alone.

I asked her, "When did this problem first come into your life?" This form of question offers an implicitly externalized, non-blaming perspective on the problem while also eliciting information that can further characterize and constrain it. She reported that it started the winter of her freshman year in college, when she started "heavily restricting" her eating and lost seven kilograms. She said she liked losing the weight, but felt "miserable" from not eating. She began eating in a pattern of restricting then bingeing, followed by excessive exercise, and later by vomiting. She said that she discovered that in doing so, she could avoid gaining weight.

We were putting together a picture of what the problem was, and in keeping our conversation—the narrative we were cocreating—close to Wonju's experience, I asked, "What should we call this problem?" Asking the patient to name the problem authorizes her as the expert on her experience of the problem and promotes greater ease in talking about the problem, especially one about which she feels shame or embarrass-ment. At first Wonju demurred, so I offered the possibility of calling it an "eating problem," but she shook her head. Bringing to mind Wonju's affiliation with nursing and the fact that she had recently taken a course on psychopathology, I then proposed "bulimia," at which Wonju looked slightly alarmed and said, "No, I don't want to think of it like that. Let's just call it 'sessions.'" Her felt experience was that it was the presence of ses-sions of purging that was the problem, and my acknowledgment of her preference helped us repair the momentary empathic failure that had resulted from my suggesting a more clinical term.

Naming a problem creates a metaphor about it that can point the way toward limiting its influence. In Wonju's case, the metaphor of "ses-sions" confined the problem to a particular duration of time and activity. The metaphor did not cast aspersions on her character or imply any fix-ity; rather, it offered the option of nonattendance, of foregoing a session. Many metaphors can be used to describe the nature of problems and which metaphor is most useful is unique to each person and situation. A problem can be seen as a constraint, imposition, or burden from which the person would like relief. Some problems are usefully defined as invi-tations or temptations that one would like to decline or habits that one wishes to change. Sometimes the problem is a rough patch in the road, a foggy bog, a mountain, a wasteland, a swamp, a toxic dump, or a desert that needs to be successfully traversed. Sometimes a problem is help-fully described as an intruder, a liar, an unwelcome guest, an unhelpful acquaintance, or a misguided friend with whom one wishes to change one's relationship. Other metaphors draw from medical language, such as seeing the problem as an illness, chemical imbalance, or diagnosis that can be treated. Preferred names and metaphors may change as treatment progresses, reflecting the patient's changing experience of the problem.[5]

Our patients sometimes arrive with non-externalized descriptions of their problems, such as "I am an anxious person." We can nonetheless develop a narrative of the problem in an externalized way, asking questions like, *What does the anxiety feel like? Is the anxiety getting you to avoid anything?* or *Are there times when the anxiety is not present?* Usually our patients welcome speaking about their concerns in an externalized way, as it frees them from experiencing their identity as indelibly infused with the problem. The difference is palpable between thinking of oneself as a depressive person or as a person dealing with a depression, as being overly perfectionistic or as someone experiencing the demands of perfectionism, or as being bulimic or hoping to forego sessions of purging. Externalization disentangles our patients' selves from their problems.

In my appointment with Wonju, my next intention was to understand the effect of the problem, the sessions, on her life. The problems our patients are facing have a range of effects on their lives, from disastrous to welcome, and we cannot know in advance what our patients' experiences are of those effects. Often it is the effects of the problem, rather that the problem itself, that are causing our patients the greatest suffering.

One resource from which I draw daily in unpacking problems is White's map for creating "a position on a problem."[6] In this map, the first task is to create an externalized, experience-near *description of the problem* in the patient's own words, as I did with Wonju earlier. Second, we seek to discover what *effects* the problem is having on the person's life—which may include aspects that are welcome as well as unwelcome. Third, we query the person as to their *assessment of the effects*; that is, to what degree those effects are wanted or unwanted. This assessment gives us grounds for asking *why* these effects are wanted or unwanted; that is, for exploring what it is to which the person gives value that the problem is affecting. This points the way toward what life might look like in the absence of the problem and how the person is already succeeding in manifesting this vision. In practice, we may do several of these tasks concurrently.

**Externalizing and Taking a Position on a Problem**

Develop an externalized, experience-near *name* and detailed *description* of the problem

Clarify the problem's *effects* on the person's life

Help the person *assess* the effects of the problem

*Compare* the effects of the problem with the person's goals and values

When I first learned this approach for understanding problems, I found it confusing and unfamiliar, entirely different from how I had been trained. But as I tried it out with patients, at first keeping a little "cheat sheet" I made on an index card close at hand, I grew increasingly comfortable with it, translating the concept into my own way of speaking and asking questions. What I like about this approach is that it first helps me understand what the problem is really like for the patient, and then it contrasts the problem with what the patient values. In others words, the problem is a problem because it is keeping someone from something they care about. Patients like this approach, because they feel I thoroughly understand their experience of the problem and also understand them better. While initially focused on the problem, this approach guides conversations in a positive direction and opens up new opportunities for cultivating narratives of strength and meaning.

I asked Wonju, "What effect are the sessions having on your life?"

"The biggest impact is that they are really exhausting," she said. Other things she didn't like was that they caused hair loss and that, now that she was living in her own apartment buying her own food, they were

## Developing the Narrative of the Patient's Relationship to the Problem

**Sample questions for eliciting an externalized, detailed, personal *description* of a problem:**

What does the depression feel like?

Where do you feel the anxiety in your body?

What are the worries getting you to avoid?

When are you noticing the perfectionism most?

When did the problem first show up?

What are the voices saying?

What should we call this problem?

What name fits this sense of unease you have been speaking of?

**Sample questions for understanding the problem's *effects*:**

What effects has the depression had on your life?

What impact do the worries have on your day-to-day life?

What has resulted from the presence of the voices?

How has the perfectionism affected your work life?

**Sample questions to help the person *assess* the effects of the problem:**

How does staying in bed all day suit you?

Do you mind not being able to drive on the highway?

How is that for you, to not get together with your friends?

Do you like spending so much time cleaning, or would you rather not?

Would it be correct to say that not enjoying your kids is the opposite of what you would want for yourself, or no?

I could imagine that someone might really not like it that even little things feel hard to do. Is that true for you?

How does it agree with you, not speaking up?

*(continued)*

**Sample questions to understand *why* the person assesses the effects of the problem as they do:**

Why would you rather not stay in bed all day?

What would be possible in your life if you were able to drive on the highway?

What does friendship mean to you?

What would you rather be doing with your time if you weren't cleaning?

What does it say about what is important to you, that you want to enjoy your kids?

If things didn't feel so hard, what would you want to make happen in your life?

Why is speaking up important to you?

causing financial strain. What she liked about the sessions was that it was "the thing that I can turn to." It was a "stress reliever" and "something I can do." She said, "I am scared to have it yanked away."

I assured her that she would get to decide the pacing of our work to reduce the impact of the sessions on her life. She then said, "I know it's bad for me. When I am in the middle of a session, in crazy mode, I am thinking to myself, this shouldn't be happening."

We went on to speak of why Wonju thought "this shouldn't be happening," of what her hopes were for herself. While she scarcely imagined it would be possible, her hopes were for a life free of sessions, in which she wouldn't be so exhausted and would have more peace of mind and energy that she could put toward the things she cared about: her career in nursing, her family, and her friendships. We paused to acknowledge the ways in which, despite the sessions, she was succeeding as a scholar, daughter, sister, and friend.

In that first meeting, we went on speak of Wonju's successes in resisting the problem, how she was "trying to quit." As a sophomore, when she was in a romantic relationship, Wonju had many days in which she did not engage in sessions, the longest for one-and-a-half weeks. She said at that time she felt "really happy," that her relationship was distracting, that she had fewer urges, and that sessions were less often on her mind. When urges did come up, she thought of how "if the person I was with found out, he might find it disgusting," and this helped her to resist.

Currently, she noted that her summer schedule was quite demanding—doing research and working as a tutor for a total of sixty hours per week—and that she was not bingeing and purging during the day, only at night. I asked if she was ever able to delay the sessions. She said, "I can delay it if I know I can do it at least once a day. If I don't do it, I feel a need to do it. I am able to not do it if I am busy. A session is both intentional and not intentional. It helps if I don't keep trigger foods around." We were putting together the story of Wonju's success in resisting the problem, and Wonju's stance was that she wanted more help in doing so. She was open to the possibility that medicine could be helpful to her.

I explained that medicines like fluoxetine could be helpful in reducing the urges to engage in sessions. We discussed the pros and cons of using fluoxetine, its side effects and potential benefits, and she elected a trial of fluoxetine, tapering up over two weeks to a therapeutic dose.

When I saw Wonju two weeks later, her expression was softer and more open. She said that she noticed a difference the week after we met, in that she felt she had "more of a choice with impulses." She offered me a small smile as she told me she had had no sessions of bingeing and purging for three days, the longest period without sessions in nearly two years. "It's not on my mind as much." She thought that the fluoxetine was probably helping her efforts to forego sessions, and the side effects of slight nausea and increased yawning were tolerable. She wanted to continue with it, as well as with psychotherapy.

One month later, she arrived for our meeting beaming. Her movements were fluid and confident as she stepped into my office and sat down on the couch. As she spoke, she warmly looked me in the eye, a smile repeatedly lighting up her whole face throughout our conversation. I smiled too. "I am definitely getting better," she said. "I have had a few lapses, but I think of them as a lapse, not a relapse." She had succeeded in limiting sessions to once or twice a week. While it was still challenging, she said, "I am stronger, I can take it on."

I asked, "How is it for you to see yourself do this?"

"It's as if a veil is lifted," she said. "There is so much more that I want to do, to enjoy. It's still hard because it's an old habit, but I will never go back."

"What lets you know that?

"It's like taking a breath of fresh air. I have achieved this recovery. I have seen that this is possible, so I can never go back to how it was."

"You have achieved this recovery and you will never go back," I repeated, nodding. "And you said there is so much more that you want to do?"

"Yes. I have been socializing much more. And when I spend time with friends, it helps me to push away the urges more. I am focusing more on what I want to do after graduation, and I am able to concentrate on my research job now."

You can hear in the preceding questions how I was fleshing out and celebrating with her the story of her recovery.

"And does 'sessions' still fit as the name for this problem or would you prefer a different name?" I asked this because I wanted to make space for her shifting relationship with problem.

"'Sessions' still fits," she said.

I then asked her about the fluoxetine. "I can feel it helping," she said. "For now it is a tool I want to use." At this point she was having no side effects. "This experience has given me a lot of insight. It's increased my interest in the field of addiction and eating disorders. And I also see how medicine can really benefit people. It's changed stereotypes I have had about using medicine."

She planned to continue psychotherapy, and expected to reduce her meetings with her therapist to every other week as she consolidated her recovery.

In our conversation above, you can hear Wonju's pride in her recovery and her sense of authority and comfort in choosing psychiatric resources to support her. She had greater awareness of her capabilities in taking on the challenge she faced and had expanded the range of what she wanted to do and to enjoy. This is what I hope for my patients. My intention is that the experience of psychiatric consultation helps to expose, circumscribe, contain, and reduce the influence of problems in my patients' lives and in their identities. In addition to offering Wonju the benefits of psycho-tropic medications, I invited her to take a perspective on the problem as separate from her sense of self and to further develop the narrative of her strengths and hopes to foster the fullest possible recovery.

## EXTERNALIZING AND UNPACKING PSYCHOSIS

What about when the problem is psychosis? When we externalize problems like paranoia or hallucinations, it serves to contain them and engages patients in discerning the nature of such problems. Patients are encouraged to develop experience-near names for problems, to clarify problems' effects, to compare those effects with their own preferences, and to reveal how problems operate.

When I was working at The Carson Center, a community mental health clinic, I met every other week with a group of five men, ages forty to fifty-five, who were dealing with schizophrenia and experi-enced ongoing or episodic psychosis. Group members named two sorts of problems: paranoia and voices. Through our conversations, George Miller, an affable, spirited member of the group, identified that the effects of the paranoia were fear and confusion. When the paranoia was active, it made him feel constantly afraid, and it was hard to figure out if that fear was warranted or not.

"Dealing with paranoia is a day's work," he said.

"Dealing with paranoia is a day's work," I repeated. The rest of the men nodded.

This was a new story. The naming and externalization of paranoia paved the way for the men to have a new relationship with it, one in which the confusing nature of paranoia was identified as such and that honored the hard work it took to differentiate realistic from unrealistic fears. Not only did this new narrative support the men's skills in managing paranoia; it also promoted a positive sense of themselves. The story of their identities changed from one of failure to one of courage, perseverance, and hard work. This new story sustained members in dealing with the expectations of others, such as those of George's father, who kept telling his son that he should just get a job.

Throughout that meeting, and during meetings over the next weeks, I repeated that sentence when we spoke about the challenges of coping with mental illness and with other's expectations, and we extended that story to dealing with other challenges: "Dealing with hearing voices is a day's work."

When psychotic symptoms are externalized, the meaning of medication changes from being about changing something wrong with the person to being a resource that might be able to help limit symptoms. In treating psychosis, it makes a great difference which stories we attend to. If we attend to the stories of determination and ingenuity in the face of excruciating symptoms and don't get distracted by claims of "craziness," we can increase our patients' ability to withstand and overcome the debilitating effects of such symptoms.

## THE STRENGTH OF IMAGINATION: A NARRATIVE APPROACH TO A DELUSION OF LOVE

A narrative approach can be used with great subtlety when dealing with meaning-laden psychotic symptoms, as in the case of Karen Larue, a down-to-earth, heavy-set thirty-eight-year-old European American woman, a single mother of two teenage children. She first consulted with me at a community mental health center after making tremendous strides of leaving an abusive relationship and stopping use of illicit drugs. She had also overcome an unrealistic obsession with a man in her neighborhood.

Karen was experiencing severe depression and flashbacks of sadistic child sexual abuse. Both her parents had been perpetrators, often giving her prized gifts after victimizing her in painful and humiliating ways. Both parents were still living, were extremely negative and blaming of her, and criticized her for leaving her violently abusive husband. It was unclear to her that she deserved to be treated with respect, and she put up with verbal abuse and at times physical violence from her fourteen-year-old son. We used fluoxetine to assist her, and although it was helpful, she continued to have ongoing suicidal impulses that she was able to resist and urges to drink and use drugs, which she was usually able to resist. She was most vulnerable to relapse when flashbacks were more active. I saw her regularly, for twenty to thirty minutes about every three weeks, treating her with antidepressant and anti-anxiety medications, while she also engaged in individual psychotherapy with a clinical social worker.

In March, about one year after I had begun working with her, Ms. Larue again began talking about Sam, a man in her neighborhood, and her current fears that he again loved her or hated her and was spreading stories about her. She declined using antipsychotic medications at that time, but when she returned in a month, she now said that she thought that this man was having contact with us at the clinic, and that he was watching her house. "At eight a.m. there was a helicopter that went by and I know he had something to do with it." It was her sense that Sam was watching over her to help her stay safe, but sometimes she worried he was planning to harm her. She said that she had tried to contact him by phone and sent him a letter, but he said that she couldn't speak with him.

I again broached the topic of antipsychotic medication, offering it as a way to decrease her sense of worry, but Ms. Larue was not interested, and in fact was angry that I was thinking about her concerns about Sam being untrue. She did not want to hear that Sam was not really in love with her. To her, the thoughts about Sam were not a problem.

I felt momentarily stuck here, because I was worried that Ms. Larue's thoughts about this man were in fact delusional, and would embarrass her and might put her in danger, and I felt a sense of responsibility to help her thoughts be based more in reality. Perhaps unpacking the meaning of Karen's thoughts about Sam might bring forward perspectives that would be useful to her.

I began by asking her about what she wanted for herself now. She spoke about trying to get her life on track, which for her included finding a satisfying relationship and staying sober. She also wanted to be able to put herself first and not capitulate to others. About Sam she said she was torn between "*let him be* versus *I wish it were me*."

I was a bit nervous about going into the "delusional material," so to speak, as my psychiatric training warned that to do so would increase it. But I also knew from my narrative training that asking questions about loved ones can be very helpful in generating positive stories in the face of despair and negative self-appraisal. So I asked her, "If you were with him, what would you be more able to appreciate about yourself?"

Karen said, "I would appreciate me for who I am. I would feel more worthwhile. He knows that I have been through a lot and survived and considers me to be a good person."

"What difference does it make to think that someone knows you have been through a lot and survived, and that you're a good person?"

"It's helpful. It would be helpful if more people knew it. They would understand me. They would know that I have nothing to be ashamed of."

These statements were the first of their kind for her. I realized that there was no one in her life past or present that had consistently related to her as if she was worthwhile. In the absence of a real source of secure relationship, she had invented one. That was the purpose of her thoughts about Sam—in the context of imagining her relationship with him, and nowhere else in her life, she could hold onto a view of herself as worthwhile, as someone who had withstood abuse for which she was not to blame and that she had nothing to be ashamed of. It was how she could think about herself if Sam loved her that allowed her to tolerate terrible flashbacks without needing to drink herself into oblivion.

We went on to speak of her ability to imagine what it would be like for her if other people knew she was a good person, and in our conversation, we were able to identify her skills of using her dreams and powerful imagination to increase her ability to put herself first and take care of herself. She found it useful to think in this way about the power and the necessity of her imagination, and by the end of our conversation, she said, "I can imagine having the willingness to take the step to look for someone who actually could be in a relationship with me and think well of me."

During the session, I wrote out a summary of our conversation for Karen, which read in part:

> You have been using your powers of having Dreams and a strong Imagination to increase your ability to put yourself first and take care of yourself. Through these abilities you are able to more strongly remember that you and other people know that you are worthwhile, that you are worthy for who you are, that you have been through a lot of terrible experiences and survived and are a good person, and that you have nothing to be ashamed of and are not to blame. You have been able to identify that your next step would be to look for someone to be in a relationship with.

My goal was to enrich and strengthen the story that she could at first only imagine, to take the story out of the delusion and make it real for her. By the end of our session, she could consider (although not entirely accept) that her hopes for a relationship with Sam were unrealistic, and identified that she wanted a real relationship. She again declined the use of antipsychotic medications.

When I saw her again three weeks later, she had completely relinquished her focus on Sam. Two months later, she continued to be free of obsessive thoughts about him, although she continued as before to cope with profound depression and posttraumatic stress disorder (PTSD) symptoms. She said, "I'm not going to live in a house like that anymore," meaning one in which she was treated with disrespect by her son. "I don't want to deal with anyone who is mean anymore." Several months later she began a program for intense treatment of substance abuse, with the intention to maintain consistent sobriety.

## SUMMARY OF EXTERNALIZING AND UNPACKING PROBLEMS

In summary, narrative psychiatry offers a framework for externalizing and unpacking a problem. Naming a problem tells a story, and I seek names that are coauthored, externalized, and experience-near to promote preferred identity conclusions. Psychiatric diagnoses sometimes meet these criteria, and biological stories about the nature of problems can be a re-authoring resource. Once the problem is named, I invite the person to take a position on it. The manifestations of the problem, which may include a story of symptoms, are exposed. The person evaluates the effects of the problem on her life based on her values and preferences. In doing so, she can compare the goals of the problem with her own goals. Then the story of successes in resisting what is problematic about the problem can be brought forward and strengthened.

In addition to understanding the effects of the problem and comparing them to the person's hopes and intentions, we can unpack problems further to reveal how they operate and the narratives that support them. Often a problem occupies a complex position in someone's life and may have both wanted and unwanted effects.

Making problems that are tenacious or disruptive to therapeutic relationships external is particularly helpful. We can avoid blaming our patients for the persistence of problems, instead identifying the source of difficulty in the problem itself, not unlike our attitude toward an aggressive cancer. For example, when we define the problem as mood volatility and intensity impinging on a person, rather than the person having a defective personality, or when we name the problem addiction rather than the person an addict, it helps us maintain a compassionate, hopeful stance that fosters nuanced, creative, and effective treatment.

## Notes

1. White, *Selected Papers,* 52.
2. Michael White, "Pseudo-encopresis: From Avalanche to Victory, from Vicious to Virtuous Cycles," *Family Systems Medicine* 2 (1984): 150–60.
3. Michel Foucault, *Madness and Civilization: A History of Insanity in the Age of Reason* (New York: Random House, 1965).
4. White, *Maps,* 9.
5. Rachael Goren-Watts demonstrated this beautifully in her research on the metaphors women use to describe their experiences of recovering from an eating disorder, "Eating Disorder Metaphors: A Qualitative Meta-synthesis of Women's Experiences" (PhD diss., Antioch University New England, Keene, NH, 2011): 88–132.
6. White, *Maps,* 54.

# CHAPTER FIVE

# Cultivating Stories of Strength and Meaning and Deconstructing Damaging Discourses

*The Course of Treatment*

Listening for narratives of strength and meaning that have not yet been told but are implicit in the patient's experience is key to the art of narrative psychiatry. In any conversation, there are many openings for finding exceptions to the activities and effects of problems. Each exception to the problem is a seed that can be cultivated into a narrative by fleshing it out with detail, linking it to other exceptions over time, and articulating the meanings that these exceptions have for the person. This new narrative offers fertile ground for freshly imagining what might be possible in the future. It sustains valued aspects of identity and points the way toward freedom from the problem.

At the same time that we are nurturing nascent stories of skill and resilience, we are also listening for narratives that fuel problems, so that they may be examined, dismantled, and replaced with narratives that support well-being. Stories that fuel problems come from many sources.

For example, someone who is dealing with depression may be influenced by a family story of being the "problem child," a local story that derides those who seek mental health treatment, and a wider cultural story that narrowly defines a successful life in terms of money. These narratives can be named and closely examined in light of the patient's own values, allowing the patient more choice over which narratives are taken up and which are set aside.

Narrative psychiatry continuously attends to the patient's social context. Often, the people who consult with us are living under the influence of cultural discourses that make negative claims about their worthiness, seek to limit their prospects, and engage them in processes of self-scrutiny that lead to anxiety or despair. By *discourses* I mean narratives and practices that share a common value.[1] These discourses include those that privilege or denigrate people on the basis of their race, gender, gender preference, sexual preference, body type, financial status, education, health, or ability. Narrative psychiatry attends to issues of power—of privilege and oppression—and deconstructs the operations of power as they influence someone's life.

This chapter demonstrates the construction of meaningful narratives and the deconstruction of damaging ones. Through sharing my work with Elena D'Amato, I show what narrative psychiatry can offer when a patient has suffered for decades from disabling symptoms. In addition, this chapter introduces the art of substantiating new narratives and identity conclusions and extending supportive communities through the use of narrative reflecting teams; that is, bringing in peers or professionals to witness and reflect in a structured way on the patient's values and skills in recovery.

## CULTIVATING STORIES OF STRENGTH AND MEANING: ELENA'S STORY

Ms. D'Amato, or Elena, as she prefers me to call her, is a warm and engaging 54-year-old Italian American woman, a registered nurse who worked professionally in her twenties. Elena is a tiny, soft-spoken, dark-haired woman, unfailingly gracious, with big, dark eyes and observant, tentative movements like a small bird. I appreciate Elena's sense of humor, talent as a baker, and ethic of care. She is happy for me to share the story of our work together in the hope that it might help others.

I met Elena eight years ago in my role as a psychiatrist at the Carson Center, a community mental health center, and we worked together for six years. She was living then with her elderly mother and her beloved dog, Bandit. At the time of our initial consultation, Elena was hearing voices throughout the day every day that harshly berated her. The voices made punishing demands, scheduling every moment of her day with household chores, requiring her to wash her hands until her skin bled, and telling her that she didn't deserve to eat. She was permitted a piece of toast for breakfast, a piece of fruit for lunch, and a salad for dinner—this despite the fact that she cooked and served a hot meal to her mother three times a day. The voices threatened Elena with even more punitive demands if she failed to meet their requirements, so she obeyed the voices "100 percent" of the time. These voices first began tormenting Elena when she was in her twenties and had been constantly present since.

The effect of the voices was that Elena's life was almost entirely taken over by them. She was unable to work professionally and her friendships atrophied. She saw a beloved aunt once a month and her brothers at Christmas. Her weight hovered at the edge of dangerously low. She was exhausted by the punishing schedule of housework. She felt it was unsafe to drive. No leisure activities were permitted her, not even half an hour of television. She was in anguish.

What might narrative psychiatry offer Elena? My first priority was to develop empathic attunement with Elena, to hear and see and feel what was most important to her and to have her feel heard and seen and felt. I heard the demands of the voices, saw who she was separate from the problems, and felt her suffering. Over time, we developed a connection we both valued.

Within this empathic field, Elena and I engaged in collaborative conversations to discover and tell stories that could open new paths to healing. We began by developing the story of her efforts to resist the voices and their demands. In any story that our patients tell of not wanting the problem they are facing is the untold story of what they do want and of their commitment to and success at making that happen, however nascently. This is one example of what Michael White calls "the absent but implicit."[2] While our patients may be focused on how they are not succeeding, their very chagrin is evidence of another narrative that is currently "absent" but can be coaxed forward. Their awareness that things could be different arises from personal knowledge of the possibility of things actually *being* different. Even simply imagining what could be different offers footing for a narrative of how they came to imagine this preferred life, what their sources of inspiration were, who might stand by them in holding a vision of this preferred future, and what preparations they may have begun to make this vision a reality.

Elena unceasingly resisted the presence of the voices. Despite the voices, she managed to skillfully care for her bedridden mother. She participated in every mental health service available. She saw a psychotherapist who offered emotional support. She had consulted with a psychiatrist for decades and took multiple medications at maximum doses. She had used psychiatric hospitalizations several times when her weight dropped to a life-threatening level. She welcomed mental health support workers into her home to monitor her medication use, take her grocery shopping, and drive her to medical appointments. All these treatments and services she found helpful, in that her suffering had been even greater without them. Highlighting Elena's efforts to resist the problem created the first sliver of space for new stories of her skill and worthiness. She had felt like a failure, and it was a new story to consider that the voices were not her fault and that she was strenuously opposing them.

Our next re-authoring project was to clarify Elena's own hopes, values, and preferences as distinct from those espoused by the voices. In the suffering-drenched experiences she described, I looked for seeds of strength and meaning to cultivate into new stories that could contribute to a more abundant sense of who she was and what might be possible in her life. In addition, doing so would allow a comparison between Elena's intentions and those of the voices, ultimately permitting a deconstruction of the values and operations of the voices that could weaken their influence. This task of clarifying Elena's hopes and values was challenging, however, because when I first met Elena, she was so fully in the grip of the voices that she experienced their perspectives as her own. She felt she was "too big" and didn't deserve to eat, and that she was unworthy and should clean all the time. The voices' cruel criticisms seemed accurate to her.

These are dicey moments in narrative psychiatry, when a person is adamant that the problem's view of things is their own. Sometimes even suggesting there is a problem is a problem. Since narrative psychiatry prioritizes what a person values over what the psychiatrist values, and seeks to create collaborative therapeutic relationships in which power disparities are minimized, there is an inherent tension in suggesting that there may be a preferable story to the one a person espouses. However, according to those who have recovered, problems such as psychosis and anorexia can sometimes separate a person from what he or she would value in the absence of the problem. Therefore, I do not accept the problem's version of a person's identity as the only version, even if an alternative story is nowhere to be seen. Rather, gentle, persistent, creative means are used to discover untold stories that are free from the influence of the problem. The imposition of the psychiatrist's perspective is in suggesting that there *is* another story; *what* that story is flows from the person's values. Cultivating the narrative of what the patient gives value to not only provides footing for diminishing the influence of psychosis or anorexia, it also guides us in developing treatment approaches that best suit the patient if psychosis or anorexia continues to dominate their experience.

In Elena's case, I sought alternative stories of her values and preferences first through asking questions about something that she felt good about, strengthening this story by asking for sensory-rich details, and extending the timeline to the past.

We had conversations that went like this:

S:   So you take care of your mother?

ELENA:  Yes.

S:  Tell me the caring things you are doing for your mother.

ELENA:  Well, I cook for her.

S:  What did you cook for her yesterday?

ELENA:  I made her eggs for breakfast.

S:  How does she like her eggs?

ELENA:  Scrambled, with toast and jam on the side.

S:  Making her eggs the way she likes them, would you say that is a sign of caring?

ELENA:  Yes.

S:  Would you say you value caring for others?

ELENA:  Yes.

S:  Who in your life knows about the ways in which you are caring for your mother?

ELENA:  I would have to say my Aunt Carla.

S:  What does Aunt Carla see, that lets her know the ways you are caring?

ELENA:  She knows I do everything for my mother. She knows that it's because of me that my mother can still be at home.

S:  Aunt Carla can see that it's because of you that your mother is still at home. Might Aunt Carla say that your care for your mother is a sign that you are a caring person?

ELENA:  I don't know. The voices, they say that I'm not doing enough.

S:  Are the voices bothering you right now?

ELENA:  Yes.

S:  That must be tiring.

ELENA:  It is.

In this conversation, you can hear how I developed a detailed account of Elena's caring actions with her mother, and then invited her to address the question of the meaning of those actions by asking if she valued caring for others.

A guide that I use in cultivating new stories of strength and meaning is the "re-authoring conversations"[3] map developed by Michael White. This map invites us to hold in awareness two aspects of experience that unfold in parallel over time: action and meaning. Each event that occurs in our lives is accompanied by the meanings we give that event. Our acts of meaning-making about our lives constitute our identities. White refers to these parallel aspects of experience as "the landscape of action and the landscape of identity."[4] In developing this idea, he drew from the psychologist Jerome Bruner, who wrote, "Story must construct two landscapes simultaneously. One is the landscape of action.... The other landscape is the landscape of consciousness: what those involved in the action know, think or feel."[5]

Events that occur in our lives that have not been noticed or ascribed meanings have little ability to contribute to the development of our identities. For example, in not ascribing meaning to what she had done to care for her mother, Elena experienced herself as someone who was not doing enough, when she was in fact solicitously caring for her mother around the clock. We can highlight neglected but significant life events and invite our patients to reflect on their meanings to facilitate identity development and to identify skills and resources they can draw on to move their lives in the directions in which they want to go.

As White puts it:

In therapeutic conversations that are oriented by re-authoring conversations, the concepts of landscape of action and landscape of identity assist the therapist in building a context in which it becomes possible for people to give meaning to and draw together in a storyline many of the overlooked but significant events of their lives. These concepts also guide the therapist in supporting people to derive new conclusions about their lives, many of which will contradict existing deficit-focus conclusions that are associated with the dominant storylines and that have been limiting of their lives.[6]

I have found it helpful to think of these as the landscape of action and the landscape of meaning, extending in parallel along a timeline that goes from the remote past, through the present, and into the future. As I create re-authoring conversations, I seek to move back and forth along this timeline by creating rich descriptions of the significant events of a person's life and linking those events to the meanings they have for the person. In this way, compelling new narratives are created.

### Sample Questions to Develop a Landscape of Action

Can you describe what you did in more detail?
What would I have seen if I could have looked in on you then?
Have you ever done that before? When? Where? What happened? Who was there?
What did you do to get ready to be able to do that?
Whose help did you enlist?
Is there another time that stands out in your memory of being able to do that?
What might someone have seen you do that exemplified that value in your life?
When was the first time you succeeded in that way?
What did you have to overcome to be able to do that?

In my preceding conversation with Elena, the questions I asked about her caring for her mother clarified the landscape of action in the new narrative we were constructing. My landscape of action questions included: *Tell me the caring things you are doing for your mother. What did you cook for her yesterday? How does she like her eggs? Who in your life knows about the ways in which you are caring for your mother? What does Aunt Carla see, that lets her know the ways you are caring?*

Landscape of action questions want to know: What did you do? How did you do it? They are designed to paint a vivid portrait of events that are relevant to the storyline at hand across different settings in the present, recent past, and remote past.

Landscape of meaning questions invite reflection about the meanings the person gives to the events that have occurred. They are evaluative and they offer opportunities for identity development. In the preceding conversation, my landscape of meaning questions included: *Making her eggs the way she likes them, would you say that is a sign of caring? Would you say you value caring for others? Might Aunt Carla say that your care for your mother is a sign that you are a caring person?*

Landscape of meaning questions want to know: What do *you* think that event says about who you are and what you care about? I added the italics in this question to emphasize that it is the *patient* who is evaluating and giving meaning to the events, not the doctor. We may have hypotheses about possible meanings that inform our questions, but our goal is for the patient to articulate his or her own meanings and values, rather than imposing our own. Not only does this honor our patients' authority and individuality, but it also generates more colorful and personal meanings that are more compelling.

We need to develop these new narratives of meaning and identity in small steps that provide a scaffold of support for the patient in reaching

---

### Sample Questions to Develop a Landscape of Meaning

What does that say about what you stand for?
What is it like to consider that you were able to do that?
Might that action be linked to a value you have?
What does it mean to you that your sister felt you were helpful then?
Is that linked to hopes or dreams you have for yourself?
Would that be evidence of a commitment you have for your life?
How is it for you to think that you were able to overcome that difficulty then?
What is that feeling of despair a testimony to?

new understandings that, while novel, ring true. One way I did this with Elena was to first invite her to ascribe meaning to one particular action, by asking, "Making her eggs the way she likes them, would you say that is a sign of caring?" Elena did. To gently extend this meaning into the arena of identity, I invited Elena to consider seeing herself as a beloved relative might see her: "Might Aunt Carla say that your care for your mother is a sign that you are a caring person?" In our early appointments, despite ample evidence, this was not a conclusion that Elena was prepared to make. You can hear how I sought to remain emotionally attuned with her by commiserating about how exhausting the voices were.

Gently, at each of our visits, I persisted in asking questions to draw forward narratives of Elena's identity that were truer to her cherished values, in contrast to the narratives of identity promulgated by the voices.

S: Would you say that people deserve to be treated with respect?

ELENA: Oh, yes.

S: Everyone, or some more than others?

ELENA: Everyone.

S: Would I have seen that value in your work as a nurse, of treating everyone with care and respect?

ELENA: Yes.

S: Yes? What would I have seen that would have let me know you value treating everyone with respect?

ELENA: Well, no matter who was assigned to me, I did my best to take care of them.

S: What kind of caring things might you do for someone?

ELENA: Well, I would be sure to check on them if they were due for their pain medicine, to see if they needed it.

In addition to clarifying Elena's values, I had a second reason to ask questions about care and respect: to create the possibility that Elena could see herself as worthy of respect. I asked, in a variety of ways over several appointments, *Since you believe everyone is worthy of respect, would you say you yourself would have to be included, that you are worthy of respect?* At first

Elena demurred, but as I gently persisted, *If you had a patient who heard voices, would you say that they should be treated with respect?* she began to consider the preposterous notion that she might be worthy of being treated with respect. This was a powerful new identity conclusion.

My third reason for asking questions about care and respect was to counter a discourse that was circulating among some of the therapists at our clinic that Elena's care for her mother was a sign of "enmeshment," whereas Elena found it to be one of the most meaningful aspects of her life, one that honored Italian American cultural traditions.

## DECONSTRUCTING NARRATIVES THAT ARE HARMFUL

My fourth reason for developing stories about care and respect was to create a starting place for Elena to begin to distinguish her values from the values enacted by the voices. The narratives that support eating disorders are particularly hard to dismantle because dieting and being thin have come to be aligned with the moral high ground in our culture, especially for women. We call declining dessert "being good" and eating a piece of cheesecake "being bad." Women who care about doing the right thing are vulnerable to buying into the story that goodness equals thinness and then taking up excessive dieting, which makes them vulnerable to developing anorexia. Once it takes hold, anorexia is a harsh taskmaster, demanding greater and greater weight loss to the point that it is life threatening. Over 5 percent of women and girls who develop anorexia die from either starvation or suicide.[7] While purporting to be the voice of righteousness and well-being, anorexia actually generates cruel lies and doesn't rest until a woman is dead.

We can unpack these tenacious discourses of "goodness" by exposing their harsh and disrespectful tone, delineating their harmful intentions, and questioning their moral claims. In doing so I am inspired by the work of Rick Maisel, David Epston, and Allison Borden in treating anorexia and bulimia, as described in their groundbreaking book, *Biting the Hand That Starves You.*[8] When the claims of moral superiority are debunked, anorexia is exposed and becomes newly vulnerable to treatment. The approach I used with Elena is applicable to anyone suffering from anorexia, since anorexia manifests by generating narratives such as "You are still too fat," and its voice, hallucinatory or not, can be identified and deconstructed. Likewise, this approach is useful for helping those dealing with other discourses of "goodness," such as those demanding excessive cleaning, washing, checking, or arranging.

So once I had helped Elena to clarify some of her values, we turned our attention to deconstructing the problem. One effective and playful way to do this is through the metaphorical strategy of personifying the problem.[9] Thinking of a problem as a person can more fully expose the manifestations and effects of a problem in a person's life, opening up more room for the person to change their relationship with the problem, and offering an opportunity to contrast the problem's effects with the person's intentions and preferences. A helpful stance to inform questioning a personified problem is one of curiosity, like that of an investigative reporter. You can ask your patient about the personified problem or you can ask him to take the role of the problem, such as "Worry," "Discouragement," "Anxiety," and so on. You can then pose questions that expose and illuminate the true intentions and inner workings of the problem. Investigating a personified problem can be useful at the first consultation, as well as in the midst of an ongoing treatment, such as Elena and I were doing.

### Sample Questions for Interviewing a Person about a Personified Problem

If this problem were a person, what name would you give it?
When is Worry most likely to show up?
What kinds of things does Anxiety do to catch your attention?
What kinds of claims does Discouragement make about your life?
What is Perfectionism's favorite way of pulling you back in when you're ignoring him?
What are Anorexia's intentions for your life?
Who in your life supports Fearfulness?
Who makes it hard for Lack-of-Confidence to have any influence?
When is Depression weakest?

Elena experienced the voices she heard as auditory hallucinations, by which I mean her perception was that she heard them like she heard my voice. I did not need to introduce the concept that we could think of the voices as people because Elena already experienced them that way. What was new to her was deconstructing the voices by thinking about their intentions and the tactics they used. Cruel voices, however, usually tend initially to become even more vociferous when they are interrogated. Gently and gradually, attending to how dangerous it was for Elena to question the voices, I asked:

S:  Would you say the voices speak to you in a caring way?

Elena:  Oh no.

S:  How would you characterize the way the voices speak to you?

ELENA:  I would say they are mean.

S:  What does it say about the voices that they would speak to you in a mean way?

ELENA:  They're not kind.

S:  Would you say that being kind is a sign of being a good friend?

ELENA:  Yes.

S:  The unkind way the voices speak to you, is that the way a good friend would speak?

ELENA:  I would have to say not.

S:  Would you say the voices are acting like a good friend to you?

ELENA:  I think they are.

S:  Even though they are mean?

ELENA:  They are trying to make me better. Keep me from getting too big.

While she wished they would go away, Elena initially said that the voices were trying to help her. But I persisted, as my intention was to be as tenacious in seeking stories that would help Elena thrive as the voices were in promoting stories that were denigrating. Gradually, over a series of appointments, I sought new ways to develop the story that the voices might not be looking out for Elena's best interests. One way I did this was by honoring her expertise and identity as a nurse.

S: As a nurse, would you say it is necessary for someone to wash their hands for ten minutes with detergent before cooking?

ELENA: I would have to say no.

S: Would you say that the advice the voices are giving about hand washing is sound from a nursing perspective?

ELENA: I would have to say no.

S: Morally, what do you think of someone who is giving advice that is not sound in terms of someone's health?

ELENA: It's not right.

S: Would you say that the voices are looking out for the best interests of your health?

ELENA: No. They say they are, but really they're not.

S: Would you say that the voices are morally in the wrong in giving harmful advice, or morally in the right?

ELENA: I would have to say that they are morally in the wrong.

We engaged in conversations like these in twenty- or thirty-minute intervals every few weeks, and gradually, over about three months, with increasing confidence, Elena told a new story: *I am a caring person who is worthy of being treated with respect. The voices are unwanted, mean, and often give bad advice. The voices claim to be good for me, but they are not.* The voices had lost their moral authority and were now open to question. This new story energized Elena and gave her hope.

Meaning is socially created and stories are strengthened by being told and retold by important figures in a person's life. If they are told only in the doctor's office, new stories are vulnerable to being overshadowed by the old problem-dominated story back home. However, in Elena's life, there were no friends or family members who could join our conversations. We invoked the presence of Elena's aunt by regularly asking questions like *Does Aunt Carla think you are worthy of being treated with respect? Would Aunt Carla favor you being addressed in such a mean way?* We also wrote new stories down on cards that Elena took home with her to reread, such as *I deserve to be treated with respect at all times.* (I actually used the piece of cardboard from the back of my prescription pads that otherwise would have gone into the recycling bin, which was nice and stiff and had a pristine white surface on one side, perfect for writing out *The voices are wrong, I don't need to scrub my hands, Just use soap and water* to be set over the sink.) I discussed our work with her long-term psychotherapist, who welcomed our approach and asked Elena about these new stories, further strengthening them.

Early in our conversations with each other, I discussed diagnostic considerations with Elena. She agreed with the diagnoses that her previous psychiatrist had proffered: schizoaffective disorder, obsessive-compulsive disorder, anorexia, and panic disorder. Despite the hegemony of *DSM*[10] diagnostic discourses in psychiatry, any diagnosis can be deconstructed.[11] We can ask, *What is helpful about using this diagnosis to describe your experience? What don't you like about using this diagnosis?* Elena felt that the diagnoses honored the severity of her problems and helped her hold onto the perspective that the voices were not real. I valued the diagnoses in that they provided me with a biological and linguistic frame for thinking about the nature of her problems and how they might respond to various treatment resources, but I resisted the pessimistic expectations of improvement associated with some of them.

As part of our re-authoring conversations, Elena and I examined her use of medicines, evaluating them according to her preferences and values. When I first met her, she was taking the antipsychotics perphenazine and risperidone to treat auditory hallucinations, fluoxetine to minimize obsessive-compulsive symptoms and depression, trazodone for insomnia, and lorazepam for anxiety. Elena was clear that she found all the medicine she was taking helpful and was reluctant to make any changes. Given the problems she described, I thought the biological effects of the medicines were a good fit, and given the severity of her symptoms, the high doses also made sense. However, she did feel tired, and I wondered if one of her medicines was contributing to that. Because of this, we changed her risperidone to aripiprazole, another antipsychotic that might be less sedating, and she reported this change was helpful. Over the next five years, as we used narrative therapy strategies to help reduce her symptoms, we tried to lower or eliminate some of her medicines, but each time Elena eventually requested that we resume them at their previous doses due to an intensification of the voices, anxiety, or insomnia.

## FINDING LOST STORIES OF STRENGTH AND MEANING

After six months of meeting together, Elena was clear that the voices were not looking out for her best interests, and she was committed to thwarting them. Our next task was to reveal their operations and dismantle them. We discovered that while the voices threatened to become even more demanding if she didn't do what they said, and did briefly intensify when she resisted them, ultimately they became less compelling. This fortified Elena in resisting them. She was newly interested in and committed to trying cognitive-behavioral treatment, and I taught her response-prevention strategies to minimize compulsive washing, cleaning, and housework.

At our meetings, we shared joy in her small steps of resistance, such as sitting for ten minutes listening to a Judy Collins song, and grief over times of resurgence of the voices. Over the next few years, we followed the percentages of her success in eating what she wanted and in resisting excessive cleaning: 5 percent, 25 percent, 30 percent, 75 percent. She added a full meal for dinner, and eventually, ice cream for dessert. After eating for the first time in ten years the little Italian cookies she baked every Christmas, she said of the voices who tried to make her feel guilty, "That shows them—they're not going to rule my life." A few months later she said, "I'm going to start taking a walk." Each day she tried to do something small that was pleasurable, such as sitting on her porch and enjoying her neighbor's flowering shrubs. Of these new developments she said, "It gives me a sense that I am worth something." She felt more capable, began driving again, and much to the surprise of her in-home support workers, cancelled their services entirely. She saw her caseworker only once every three months. She spoke with more confidence and humor in our meetings, which became less frequent. After three years of working together using narrative psychiatry, she experienced a four-month period in which the voices were entirely absent, she was not engaging in compulsive cleaning or washing, and she was eating full meals. She reconnected with an old friend from nursing school. We celebrated these developments with joy and relief. Then Bandit died, and a few months later, Aunt Carla died. All of Elena's symptoms returned in full force.

I grieved with Elena the loss of a dear relative who had been a consistent, life-long source of loving support, and of her dog, who had been her constant companion. We also grieved the return of the voices and their demands. However, I was not discouraged in that I knew that the story of Elena's worthiness and of the illegitimacy of the voices was still present, if obscured, and could be re-evoked.

Here is part of a conversation we shared during this time, which Elena gave me permission to tape. It is edited for brevity and clarity. Notice how we discovered a small moment of resistance to the problem and strengthened it into an inspiring story by developing detail, naming themes, finding similar examples from the remote past, invoking important figures from her life, and anticipating how she can apply these new understandings to dealing with her problem.

At the start of this conversation, Elena is subdued and even more soft-spoken and tentative than usual. She spoke about having a hard time stopping the voices, how they started waking her up in her sleep, and that she felt she was losing her mind.

ELENA: I am wondering, do I really feel this way or do I just think I feel this way. I need some extra help and I am not sure what I need. I talked to Chris [her case worker] about it.

S: You're feeling you could us some extra help, and you and Chris talked about that?

ELENA: Yes.

S: And what did you come up with?

ELENA: Well, she said she said she would call more on the phone, and instead of hiding how I felt, she wanted me to—even if I didn't think it was right or not—to tell her.

S: Uh huh, and so, is that something that you thought would be helpful, or you thought was worth a try?

ELENA: Yes.

S: And would that be a new step for you, to tell her how you were really feeling?

Elena: Yes.

S: And your hopes, in terms of telling her how you were really feeling, what were your hopes for what might happen?

Elena: That whatever is inside of my head will…will stop.

S: Mmm hmmm. And what does it take for you to actually share with her what you are really feeling? Were you able to actually do that when you met with her this last time?

Elena: Not at first. But eventually.

S: And how did you get yourself to do that?

Elena: I think I was feeling so bad that I…I needed to find out what was real or not….

S: Mmm hmm.

Elena: And I usually don't try to tell people how I feel, you know, everything's usually okay.

S: You mean that is what you usually say?

Elena: Yes.

S: You usually say everything is okay. But this time you made a different choice, because you really wanted things to change for you?

Elena: Yes.

S: You really wanted to feel better. Was there a way, despite feeling confused and depressed, that you held onto the hope that things could be different for you?

Elena: Yes.

S: And where did that hope come from, the hope that things could be different for you?

Elena: Um, because I…I, um, always seem to be able to fight back.

S: Uh huh.

Elena: (smiles.)

S: That's a strong statement, that you always seem to be able to fight back. You've seen yourself fight back. Have you had to fight back other times?

Elena: Yes.

S: Would you say that it's something you have had to do lots of times?

ELENA: Yes. (nods)

S: Lots of times. Is there another time that stands out for you of fighting back? When you had to fight back?

ELENA: I...I'm not sure. Like when I went to school I was in the slow class, and I had to go to summer school every year, and, but I kept trying and I think I did pretty good, because I went and got my degree and everything.

S: Your bachelor's degree.

ELENA: Yes.

S: Uh huh. So that really took a bit of a fighting spirit, would you say, to keep going through school? And take summer school and everything?

ELENA: Uh huh.

S: And who supported you in having that kind of fighting spirit?

ELENA: I think my family.

S: Your family? Who in particular?

ELENA: My mother.

S: And how would you see her supporting your fighting spirit?

ELENA: She would encourage me to, you know, do what I wanted to do but make sure it wasn't too much.

S: She would encourage you to do what you wanted but not do too much. Can you give me a specific example of when she encouraged you?

ELENA: Well like when I went to nursing school, I started out in a diploma program, but I always wanted to advance myself, but I had a hard time with learning things, but I had the chance to go for my bachelor's degree, and I did, you know, good, and then I went to UMass and I struggled but I have my master's degree.

S: And your mother encouraged you. What might she say to you?

ELENA: She used to tell me, "You don't have to be the best."

S: Uh huh.

ELENA: You know. I felt like I had to do better so they would be proud of me.

S: Uh huh. For your family…

ELENA: Yes.

S: …your mother.

ELENA: Because they never got the opportunity…

S: To go to college. So what do you think it meant to your mother that you actually stayed in there and used your fighting spirit to get a bachelor's degree and then a master's degree? What do you think it meant to her?

ELENA: I think it meant a lot. I think she was happy that, you know, I made it as far as I did.

S: How would you say do you think it made her feel as your parent?

ELENA: Proud.

S: Proud. And would you say that it made her feel good about herself as a parent that a child she raised could have these opportunities and stick with it?

ELENA: Yes.

S: Okay. So this legacy of a fighting spirit is part of what you are drawing on now?

ELENA: Uh huh.

S: To share with Chris about how you are really feeling, and that things really are pretty tough right now?

ELENA: Yes.

S: And are you drawing on it now to talk to me about how tough things are right now?

ELENA: Yes.

S: And saying things are extra tough, and that you need extra help?

ELENA: I feel like I can tell you how I really feel.

S: You do. And what lets you feel like you can do that?

ELENA: Because you accept me no matter what, you know, if I'm doing good or doing bad.

S: Uh huh. It feels…we have set up our relationship where it feels comfortable for you to say whatever is happening.

ELENA: Uh huh.

S: So did you and Chris come up with some things that might be supports right now?

ELENA: Yes, she is helping me figure out what is real and what isn't real.

You can hear how I lingered with Elena in speaking about the new step she was taking in telling her caseworker, Chris, about how she was really feeling. These tiny positive moments are seeds of strength that can be cultivated. In the midst of a dramatic recurrence of harsh voices and Elena feeling that she was losing her mind, this small step might have been missed, or glossed over, but in narrative psychiatry these tiny movements and intentions are noticed, named, and nurtured into narratives that point the way toward recovery and offer inspiration for the journey.

In developing the narrative of her new step, I first spoke with Elena about what she did in speaking with Chris (landscape of action), asking, *You're feeling you could use some extra help, and you and Chris talked about that? And what did you come up with?* When she said that she was going to tell Chris what she was really feeling, I asked her to put meaning and intentionality to what she did (landscape of meaning), asking, *And would that be a new step for you, to tell her how you were really feeling? What were your hopes for what might happen?*

I then returned to asking more about what she did (landscape of action again): *Were you able to actually do that when you met with her this last time? And how did you get yourself to do that?* And then I segued into asking again about the meaning of what she did: *Was there a way, despite feeling confused and depressed, that you held onto the hope that things could be different for you? And where did that hope come from, the hope that things could be different for you?* Here is where Elena attributed further meaning to the new step she was taking, making a statement of identity: *I always seem to be able to fight back.*

We were then able to develop the narrative of how she was able to fight back, tracing its history from her infancy through her college years.[12] I asked her first for the details of events that illustrated the theme of fighting back, and then I asked her to put meaning to those events through the eyes of her mother: *What do you think it meant to your mother that you actually stayed in there and used your fighting spirit to get a bachelor's degree and then a master's degree?* Asking patients to see themselves through the eyes of a loved one offers additional substance to new identity considerations. One shortcoming in this conversation is how I used the phrase "fighting spirit" without checking out with Elena if that was a good fit. It would have been better to stick with her phrase "fighting back" because using the patient's language honors her authority and creates a more compelling, experience-near narrative.

After developing the narrative of Elena's commitment to fight back, I brought the story back around to the initiatives that she was taking in the present and would take in the near future: *So this legacy of a fighting spirit is part of what you are drawing on now? To share with Chris about how you are really feeling? And are you drawing on it now to talking to me about how things are tough things are right now?* Elena then made a beautiful statement about her experience of our connection: *I feel like I can tell you how I really feel.* I lingered here a bit, asking, *And what lets you feel like you can do that?* so as to deepen her sense of our connection and her awareness of how she knows what she knows. In response, she furthered the narrative about our connection, saying, *Because you accept me no matter what, if I'm doing good or doing bad.* I was warmed by her words and glad that we had been able to create the kind of collaborative connection and emotional attunement to which they referred.

## NARRATIVE REFLECTING TEAMS

Ten days after this conversation, with Elena's permission, I shared her story and the videotape of this session at a narrative psychiatry workshop that I led, inviting the participants to be witnesses in the reflecting team style of narrative psychotherapy.[13] Narratives are strengthened and new identity conclusions are substantiated when they are shared by others. There are many ways we can bring additional witnesses in to hear and retell the healing stories that our patients develop. Family members and friends can be invited in to hear about new life initiatives and extend those narratives with fresh examples and innovative meanings. Others who have overcome similar problems may welcome the chance to be helpful and be welcomed by patients to hear and honor the story of their journey. And other professionals can generate rich retellings of our patients' new narratives that are moving and inspiring.

Of course, not all retellings of our patients' stories honor them or help support their new initiatives toward well-being. Unless specifically guarded against, the most likely thing is for the familiar problem-dominated narrative to be repeated. To support our intention for nurturing new, preferred narratives, we can draw on the reflecting team practices first developed by Tom Anderson[14] and further refined by Michael White.[15] Developing these practices over decades of experience, White discovered that patients find it most helpful when witnesses respond to the following kinds of questions: *What words that the person said stayed with you? Why are these expressions meaningful to you personally? What image of the person do those words inspire? How did hearing this person's story change you?* After telling her story, the patient is invited to listen in on the conversation between her doctor and the witnesses, who speak about the patient in the third person. This frees the patient from the obligation to respond to what is said, allowing her the privilege of simply taking in what the witnesses are saying. Once the witnesses have finished speaking, then the patient is invited to reflect on what was said, speaking about what stayed with her and why, and what difference it makes to her.

So at the workshop, I proposed that the participants write responses to Elena that included what words stayed with them and why, what

---

**Questions to Guide Reflection by Witnesses**

What words that the person said stayed with you?
Why are these expressions meaningful to you personally?
What image of the person do those words inspire?
How did hearing this person's story change you?

image of her they inspired, and how hearing her story changed them. Here is one response by a therapist who has given permission to share it with you:

> Your courage stood out for me. My grandfather struggled with voices and his life was very painful and dark. He was someone I loved very much and I wish there could have been treatment that eased his struggle. I guess I felt he gave up in ways, and I saw in you a courage to go on, despite the confusion and the pain. My image of you is of a gentle warrior. I do yoga and the warrior poses are of strength, relaxation and balance. How did hearing your story change me? It gave me more understanding of how hard my grandfather might have worked to resist the voices.

I brought eleven similar letters back to Elena and we read them together. She wept with emotion, to hear how her story moved and inspired others. The letters became one of her most treasured possessions, and over the years, rereading them was one of her most effective strategies. Over the next six months, Elena again reclaimed her life from the demands of the voices. At times of loss the voices have surged up and tried new ways to prevail, but Elena has successfully constrained them, and in the last few years she has enjoyed longer and longer periods in which she is free to live as she prefers.

## SUMMARY

In practicing narratively, our ears are continuously tuned to listen for narratives of strength and meaning that haven't yet been told but are implicit in the patient's experience. Often people have skills and commitments of which they are not fully aware, such as Elena, who identified her commitment to hold onto hope and to fight back to create the life she wanted to be living. Throughout treatment, we can identify seeds of strength and coauthor new stories that orient our patients to their values and abilities and inspire them to take actions that help them recover and thrive. In doing so, we can strive to honor what our patients value, rather than imposing our own values. Likewise, we can attend to the narratives that are influencing our patients, deconstructing those that are antagonistic and cultivating those that contribute to a positive sense of identity. In Elena's case, resisting the voices and their demands meant dismantling the notion that thinness equaled goodness, and substantiating the story of her worthiness, courage, and success—a story that was further developed, circulated, and strengthened by witnesses offering their reflections.

I have found my work with Elena to be among the most meaningful of my career. It showed me that loving perseverance in applying narrative psychiatry can help pave the way for someone to experience long stretches of peacefulness and contentment after decades of unremitting torment. Now you, dear reader, are part of her story, too, as well as the stories of all the patients described in this book; and if you wish, you may send me your reflections of which words of theirs stayed with you, why those words are meaningful to you personally, what image of the person they evoke, and what difference it has made to you to hear their story, and I will be sure my patients get them.

## ELENA'S REFLECTIONS

Elena and I ended our work together two years ago when I left the Carson Center to take my current position at the University of Massachusetts–Amherst, and we were both happy to be back in touch when I sent her this chapter to read.

Elena offered the following reflection on it:

Dr. Hamkins really changed my life and made it worth living. To this day, I still use what she taught me and it has helped me through some difficult times. My mother has since passed away and I had a hard time dealing with it and was hospitalized for a month, but

Dr. Hamkins gave me the knowledge and support that I used to get me through. To this day, I still use the cards she made for me to read to fight the voices and I read them daily and they give me the strength to keep fighting and feel deserving. I still have the letters she shared with me from the participants in the lecture she gave and read them also. I have never had someone who influenced my life so positively.

In her letter to me, she also included a new development in her life:

I just have to tell you, I adopted a cat about a month ago from the shelter. They did not know much about him, but he was found wandering the streets. You will never guess the name they gave him. It was Bandit, so I kept it the same. My Bandit has come home to me.

## Notes

1. Rachel Hare-Muston, "Discourses in the Mirrored Room: A Postmodern Analysis of Therapy," *Family Process* 33 (1994): 35.
2. White, "Re-engaging with History," 35.
3. White, *Maps,* 61.
4. Ibid., 83.
5. Jerome Bruner, *Actual Minds, Possible Worlds* (Cambridge, MA: Harvard University Press, 1987), 14.
6. White, *Maps,* 83.
7. Laird Birmingham et. al., "The Mortality Rate from Anorexia Nervosa," *International Journal of Eating Disorders* 38 (2005):143–6, doi:10.1002/eat.20164.
8. Richard Maisel, David Epston, and Alison Borden, *Biting the Hand that Starves You* (New York: W.W. Norton, 2004).
9. Sallyann Roth and David Epston, "Consulting the Problem about the Problematic Relationship: An Exercise for Experiencing a Relationship with an Externalized Problem," in *Constructive Therapies*, vol. 2, ed. Michael Hoyt (New York: Guilford, 1996), 148–62.
10. American Psychiatric Association, *Diagnostic and Statistical Manual of Mental Disorders*, 4th ed., Text Revision (Washington, DC: American Psychiatric Association, 2000).
11. Michael White, *Re-authoring Lives: Interviews and Essays* (Adelaide, Australia: Dulwich Centre Publications, 1995), 19.
12. In this case, Elena brought forward a metaphor of fighting back that she found helpful, but Michael White (*Maps*, 34–37) reminds us to avoid entrenchment in any one

metaphor, especially black-and-white, adversarial metaphors as they can become draining and limiting. Listening for other metaphors of success opens up possibilities for a range of energizing narratives that can contribute more richly to well-being. For example, in her reflection upon this chapter, in addition to "fighting back," Elena describes "feeling deserving" as a positive development, a metaphor that could open up refreshing new possibilities for identity development and positioning herself relative to the voices.

13. White, *Maps*, 165–218.
14. Tom Anderson, "The Reflecting Team: Dialogue and Meta-Dialogue in Clinical Work," *Family Process* 26 (1987): 415–28.
15. White, *Maps*, 197.

# CHAPTER SIX

# Collaborating in Choosing Treatment Options

## Medicines and Other Psychiatric Resources

In practicing narratively, the doctor and patient can examine together what the doctor's kit of psychiatry might have to offer in light of the values and preferences of the person seeking consultation, which authorizes the patient as the arbiter of what is helpful and what is not. Narrative psychiatry holds the perspective that while the doctor may have specialized knowledge about treatments, the patient is the expert on his or her life, and medicine or other treatments can be evaluated according to the values and preferences of the patient. In its nuanced approach to effective collaboration, narrative psychiatry offers ways to more fully manifest the intentions of the mental health recovery movement. This chapter will show how to collaborate with patients in considering and choosing among psychiatric resources such as psychotropic medications. In doing so, it will touch on the range of competing discourses about psychiatric treatments that may be influencing our patients and us.

The story we have come to hold about who the patient is and what the problem is determines the therapeutic options we consider. All the skills described in the previous chapters—emotional attunement; developing a rich portrait of who the person is separate from the problem; clarifying the patient's vision for his or her life; creating an externalized, experience-near description of the problem and its effects; and cultivating a narrative of how the person is resisting the problem and how that is linked to personal hopes and values—are prerequisites for being able to collaboratively consider which resources might best meet the patient's needs. From our initial consultation on, we cultivate very different stories about the patient and the problem depending on the questions we ask—or don't ask. Creating narratives that articulate our patients' personal experiences of their problems and that honor their resiliencies, skills, and preferences sets the stage for considering treatments that will be most effective and life enhancing.

When we have a collaborative therapeutic stance, we can look side by side with our patients at the wealth of treatment options that might be helpful and weigh the pros and cons together. Whether we are considering mindfulness practices, somatic experiencing, family therapy, dialectical behavior therapy, an exercise regimen, partial hospitalization, peer-led advocacy groups, or psychotropic medications, we can work with our patients to help them determine the approach with which they feel most comfortable. Once we clarify our patient's wishes, we can offer the preferred treatment ourselves or facilitate a referral to someone who can.

Of course, psychiatric treatments are just a fraction of the resources that people draw on to take steps toward their hoped-for futures. Families, religious communities, cultural centers, friendship networks, and other relationships that are integral to the fabric of people's lives are the foundations of support and point toward culturally syntonic resources for responding to challenges—such as Vanessa in chapter 2 finding a "gang of friends" who support and inspire her. In cultivating stories of strength and meaning, we are seeking to make these relationships and resources more apparent and easier to access.

In addition, advocacy and peer support networks such as Active Minds,[1] the National Alliance on Mental Illness,[2] the International OCD Foundation,[3] and the Depression and Bipolar Support Alliance[4] offer support and advocacy for people who identify as dealing with a mental health challenge. Other organizations such as the Hearing

**Sample Questions for Collaboratively Considering Psychiatric and Recovery Resources**

Response-prevention strategies and medicine both can be helpful in minimizing urges to go overboard cleaning. Would you be interested in hearing more about either of them?

There are several strategies that can help reduce the frequency and intensity of anxiety attacks. Would you like me to tell you about some of them?

Some people have found a therapy called somatic experiencing to be helpful in getting over anxiety that stems from a car accident. Does that interest you?

In addition to psychotherapy, some people have found it helpful to also use medicine to help them reduce the torment of depression. Is that something you want to consider, or no?

At times like these, many people have found it helpful to get a lot more support, such as attending an intensive outpatient program that meets five days a week. What do you think about that option?

Some people who hear voices find it helpful to meet with others who are having similar experiences. Would you like to hear more about that possibility?

There is a national organization with a chapter here on our campus called Active Minds that works to support mental health and reduce stigma. Does that interest you?

Voices Network[5] and the Icarus Project[6] and events sponsored by the Mad Pride movement[7] offer support and advocacy to people who identify as dealing with extreme or distressing experiences, who may or may not prefer to describe their experiences in psychiatric terms. In collaboratively creating plans for recovery, we can consider all of these resources, according to the preferences of the person seeking consultation.

# NARRATIVE PSYCHOPHARMACOLOGY

One resource that many of our patients find a compelling option is psychotropic medication. Narrative practices are wonderfully conducive to life-enhancing psychopharmacology. Psychopharmacology informed by narrative psychiatry combines the resources of re-authoring conversations and psychotropic medicines. It seeks to understand the relationships among the body, the mind, well-being, and medicine, and stories about the body, the mind, well-being, and medicine.

The efficacy of psychotropic medications is currently in contention both outside and within the field of psychiatry. Irving Kirsch,[8] a psychologist, found in his review of a range of typical short-term psychiatric drug studies that antidepressant medicines are no more effective than placebos for mild to moderate depression. The investigative reporter Robert Whittaker[9] went further, making a case that the medicines commonly prescribed for anxiety, depression, and psychosis are actually making people worse, and cites evidence that people with psychosis in countries where the use of psychotropic medications is rare have better outcomes than countries where it is common, such as the United States. He notes that the number of people in the United States receiving disability benefits for mental health concerns has dramatically increased over the decades in which psychotropic medicines have become popular, implying a link; others, however, ascribe the dramatic increase in the number of people receiving federal disability payments over the last thirty years to the decrease in the number of families on welfare and the increase in unemployment.[10] The work of psychiatrist Jaako Seikkula has demonstrated that gentle family therapy and no or minimal use of antipsychotic medications has improved long-term outcomes for patients experiencing initial episodes of psychosis.[11] Many people have found that the negative effects of psychotropic medicines outweigh any benefits and eschew their use.

At the same time, others swear by them. They report that psychotropic medicines have been an invaluable resource that help relieve their suffering—similar to how many people feel about Novocain when they have a cavity filled or ibuprofen for chronic arthritis. Placebo effects do not account for patients' experience that some antidepressants work well in relieving their symptoms while others do not. Patients with the most severe symptoms are most likely to be prescribed medications. When patients experience the return of symptoms when they stop their medicines, it may mean that the medicines are making them worse, or it may mean that the medicines are helpful and necessary.

What we know about psychotropic medicines and the neurochemical functioning of the brain is tiny compared with what we do not know. This means that judiciousness and transparency are called for in offering our patients the resource of psychotropic medicines, including a willingness to speak frankly about their limitations and potential negative effects. It also behooves us to have more than just drugs in our psychiatric toolkit. The practices of narrative psychiatry are tools that I have found particularly helpful.

Medicines have both rhetorical and non-rhetorical effects. That is, a person's experience of using a medicine is constituted both by stories about the medicine and by the physical effects of the medicine on their body. I think of the placebo effect as a narrative effect; in other words, the benefits that patients get from the act of taking a medicine that may not offer any biological benefits are due to the story they hold that the medicine will be helpful to them. When my patients who have had a prompt positive response to a medicine say, "I think I am having a placebo effect," I generally respond, "Yes, you undoubtedly are, and I am glad you are, because you are feeling better, *and* you may also be having a positive biological effect, too." The reality is that, in practice, it is almost impossible to know for any given person whether the benefit he or she is experiencing is placebo or biological.

Like other kinds of re-authoring conversations, narrative conversations about medicines can move between landscapes of action (the physical effects of a medicine) and landscapes of meaning (the meaning the person ascribes to the effects). Patients are authorized to evaluate effects of medicine in light of their own values and preferences. Ultimately, the most important piece of data about a drug is the patient's own experience in taking it.

Given the range of mental health challenges our patients face, the range of discourses about those challenges, the range of psychotropic medicines available, and the range of discourses about these medicines, practicing narrative psychopharmacology can be complex. Because we work with our patients to find medicines that meet their needs and enhance their lives, it is often joyful.

## NARRATIVE PSYCHOPHARMACOLOGY IN ACTION: ALEXIS'S STORY

We can see both complexity and joy in my work with Alexis Gray, a bright spark of a young woman with a dry sense of humor and a frank, informal manner. She was in her early to mid-twenties over the six years I worked with her. Of European American ancestry, Alexis swung her stiff right leg in an energetic gait down the hall to my office for our monthly meeting and gazed out at me forthrightly through thick glasses as she made animated conversation. At the time we are picking up her story, she had been consulting with me about psychiatric medicines for several years as part of her efforts to move her life in the direction in which she preferred.

At that time, Alexis was focused on building a foundation for the future she wanted, which included getting a formal education, becoming a counselor, becoming a parent, maintaining her health, and having a loving community of friends. Over the years I had worked with her, I came to appreciate how her values included care for all people, with a particular respect for people such as herself who have survived serious trauma and may be coping with mental health problems. I saw how she valued egalitarian relationships among doctors and those who consult with them. Alexis was an expert about consulting with doctors, as she had been doing so since early childhood, when she had been in a serious car accident that originally left her unable to talk or walk. She had consulted regularly with psychiatrists since she was ten, including during several psychiatric hospitalizations.

Among other challenges she was then facing, Ms. Gray was trying to prevent anxiety from making a comeback in her life, in the context of her grandmother dying and her father subsequently holding her mother at gunpoint for three hours before being arrested and hospitalized. In this context, Alexis was concerned that she was overusing lorazepam (Ativan).

S: How much have you been taking?

ALEXIS: Four a day.

S: That's quite a lot, twice as much as we had talked about.

ALEXIS: I know. I don't like taking it.

S: One of my concerns is that Ativan is addictive, and if you take it every day, it will stop working as well.

ALEXIS: Then I want to stop it. I'm sorry, but you know I hate taking medicine.

S: I do know. It's fine to stop the Ativan, but it's best to stop it gradually so you don't have withdrawal effects. What I would recommend is going back down to two tablets a day for a week, then one tablet at bedtime for a week, then a half a tablet at bedtime for a week. How does that sound?

ALEXIS: Good.

S: So let's talk about what else might be helpful at keeping the anxiety out of your life.

As I discussed the lorazepam with Alexis, many discourses were influencing our conversation. The stories of the benefits of re-authoring conversations of narrative psychiatry led me to consider what landscapes of meaning and action were influencing Alexis's experience of her life, and to offer opportunities for her to construct stories that helped her experience her life as she preferred. The story of her ingenuity and determination in resisting stress was one such story.

Another discourse at play is the psychopharmacologic story about the risks and benefits of medicines like lorazepam. Risks include the potential for addiction and sedation, while benefits include the effect of lorazepam on gamma-aminobutyric acid receptors in the brain, which leads to a temporary enhancement of physical and mental calm. I find the medical story of lorazepam to be useful and its warning about addiction is in line with Alexis's values. However, its biological purview is narrower than the aspects of life and means of resistance that Alexis finds important. She prefers to minimize the use of medicine and to focus on other ways of achieving well-being. The psychopharmacologic story also has an individualistic purview; that is, it sees the problem as the person having excessive anxiety. In contrast, a story with a broader scope based on values such as social justice might focus on how anxiety may be supported by the pressures contemporary society puts on its less privileged and more vulnerable members.

In considering the stories that are evoked in consultation, I find it helpful to remain aware that the dilemma continuously exists in narrative psychiatry that the opinions and values of the doctor may become overly centered when discussing the risks and benefits of medicines. This dilemma is minimized when we have cocreated a clear understanding of what the patient's values, preferences, and intentions are. Then in conversation together, the therapist and the person can compare the effects of a medicine to the person's preferences. Offering ideas about medicine tentatively or offering a range of possibilities can allow someone more freedom to choose what he or she truly prefers. Sometime when I offer possibilities, people consulting with me say, "You're the expert, you tell me what I should do." I generally reply, "I know about the medicine, but you're the expert on your life." Then I pose a few more questions that help to clarify what their values are and what they hope the medicine might do for them, and with this additional scaffolding, their own preferences become more available to be voiced in our conversations. Alexis had made it clear that the risk of addiction and the overuse of medicine were against her preferences, and I offered information geared to that preference.

Alexis consulted with me again a month later. She noted that she continued to feel stressed and was grieving the death of her grandmother, which evoked for her the deaths of her sisters. She was succeeding in managing the anxiety and had stopped daily use of lorazepam, using it only once every few weeks.

Four months later, Alexis came in reporting that there was a "lot of excitement" because she had started school and was working on her General Educational Development certificate, or GED, which would allow her to apply to college. Here are some of the things she said during that conversation with me:

> I've had a lot of excitement lately because I started school to work on my GED…. School has been pretty good, but it's hard. I'm getting one-on-one tutoring which helps. It'll take me two years to finish…. Depression is hitting me because I'm getting memories of all the times that people told me it would be impossible for me to get my GED. Plus I'm dealing with riding the bus, which is anxiety provoking because the last time I rode a bus, when I got off I was raped…. I carry Ativan with me, but I haven't needed to take it. I've been able to cope with the anxiety without it.

At our next meeting a month later, she said:

> I'm not using the Ativan, but I am able to ride the bus anyway. The bus makes me nervous, but my motivation to get my education is stronger than my fear of riding the bus. I don't like using the Ativan because it makes me tired during the day…. I got an EEG [electroencephalogram] done. It showed general slowing but no signs of seizures. My neurologist isn't concerned about it…. My concentration is bad, though, and I think it would really be helped by Ritalin. I have always had concentration difficulties but I have never been diagnosed with bona fide ADD.

When Alexis was five years old she was hit by a car and sustained serious brain injury. Following the brain injury, she had a severe tremor, constriction of her right hand, an uneven gait, and challenges to her thinking and sensations. In consultation with her neurologists, two years earlier she had had a deep brain stimulator placed that markedly reduced the severity of the tremor.

What are the narratives that emerge in hearing about Alexis and her request to use methylphenidate (Ritalin)?

For me, a primary narrative on which I focused was the story of Alexis's values and commitments to having the life she wanted, including getting an education, working as a psychotherapist, becoming a parent, having friends, and minimizing the ways in which physical and mental health challenges are constraining her. I was moved by her commitments to overcome fear to be able to ride the bus to school and by her efforts to educate herself despite neurological challenges, like brain wave slowing. The image that her daring and commitment brought forward for me is of Alexis digging out from under the rubble of several traumatic earthquakes that have rocked her life, and using those stones and others to build a beautiful home for her life. She inspired me in my work with others to listen even more carefully for hopes and dreams, knowing that dreams can be nurtured and can come true even when challenges seem insurmountable. Now she was facing the challenge of concentration difficulties.

A relevant medical narrative is the meaning given to slowed brain waves measured on the EEG. Slowed brain waves are usually associated with someone who is experiencing severe cognitive difficulties, such as from Alzheimer's disease or encephalitis. Alexis has found the following to be a useful story: a problem that is constraining her is that her brain was injured years ago and is now is functioning in a way that is making it difficult for her to think, remember, and concentrate.

A psychopharmacologic narrative is the effect methylphenidate might have on Alexis's brain, possibly leading to better concentration and cognitive clarity. Methylphenidate is understood to be a mild stimulant of the brain as a whole, but its exact mode of action is not known. What is known is that many people who take methylphenidate say they can concentrate better. In this, methylphenidate is similar to caffeine, but more powerful. Methylphenidate has known dangers that include seizures, especially in people who have had brain injury or brain surgery (Alexis has had both). It also causes appetite suppression and can be addictive. Because of these dangers, methylphenidate prescribing and use is closely monitored in the United States.

A social justice narrative is how the responses of children and adults to the demands of modern society have been harmfully pathologized, and how methylphenidate and other stimulant medications have been promoted as a solution for what are seen as culturally generated problems, when children and adults would be better served by other means. A related story is how certain educational and career achievements have been harmfully reified as the necessary for a successful life, while other aspects of life, such as values, love, and relationships, have been less honored.

A performance-enhancement narrative asks, if methylphenidate improves cognitive performance, why not use it?[12]

In light of all these stories, how should one proceed in trying to practice narrative psychopharmacology? Far from being unusual, many psychopharmacologic consultations evoke a similar range of discourses. Our work is most challenging when discourses we value contradict one another, as they do here.

Alexis was clear she wanted to try methylphenidate to help her reach goals that she had had to persist against great odds to imagine might be possible for her, and this was an important consideration for me as her consultant. Through our conversations about her hopes and dreams, we were coauthoring her definitions of a life worth living, implicitly counteracting damaging discourses that disparaged the abilities and worth of people with brain injuries as well as those that overemphasized achievement and normalcy.

As I considered all these narratives, what stood out for me was the strong possibility that methylphenidate would biologically increase Alexis's ability to concentrate and think clearly. In seeking help to better organize her thoughts, resist impulsive actions, and reduce depression and emotional distress, Alexis had already tried many different kinds medicines, of which none were consistently helpful. She had never had problems with addiction or high use of substances, so I felt the risk of addiction for Alexis was low. However, I was concerned that she might be at risk of seizures due to her traumatic brain injury and brain surgery.

Furthermore, Alexis explicitly asked to try methylphenidate. I value working against power imbalance in psychopharmacologic consultation. A dilemma is that a person can only get certain medicines if a doctor writes them a prescription. I endeavor to have prescriptions I write lead to desired biological effects, to support a person living their life as they prefer, and to contribute to preferred identity conclusions. Any time a person is considering taking a medicine that is new to them, the risks, benefits, and side effects are theoretical and not experience-near. I see it as my job to explain as clearly as possible these positive and negative effects, so that a person can make a decision about a medicine in light of his or her own values. It is also my job to refrain from prescribing medicines that I believe will be harmful for a particular person, even if they request them. I see refraining from prescribing potentially harmful medicines as analogous to refraining from engaging in potentially harmful psychotherapeutic processes, even if a person requests those. In both instances, I am striving to be "influential but decentered,"[13] using my skills to offer therapeutic resources that I think will be most helpful to a person in light of their preferred identity.

At times, helping a person experience a preferred identity is best supported by honoring their request for medication. Such was my conclusion here with Alexis, for all the reasons offered above—as long as her neurologist thought it was reasonably safe. We checked with him, and he said that there were no dangerous risks for her in trying methylphenidate. So we gave it a try, starting with a low dose of 5 mg twice a day.

Two weeks later we met again.

S:   Did you try the Ritalin?

ALEXIS:  Yes I did.

S:   So what do you think?

ALEXIS:  I'm having no side effects whatsoever, and a little bit of a positive effect.

The conversation began with me authorizing Alexis as the person with the power to choose whether or not to actually take the medicine we had discussed at the previous appointment. The question *Did you try the Ritalin?*

honored her agency and did not presuppose that the answer would be yes. The choice to take or not take a medicine is personal and is linked with the values and preferences a person holds for his or her life. The concept of compliance in narrative psychiatry is applied opposite its meaning in psychiatry-as-usual. The relevant question is: *How well is the doctor complying with the person's preferences in offering medicine options?* For Alexis, trying methylphenidate was a good match with her preferences.

---

**Sample Questions to Collaboratively Evaluate the Helpfulness of Psychotropic Medicine**

Did you decide to try the medicine?
What has it been like?
What do you think about its effects?
How does that suit you?
What exactly has been positive about it?
What negative effects are you experiencing?
Does it seem to you that the benefits of the medicine outweigh
    the negative effects?
What questions do you have about this medication?
What are your thoughts about using this medicine?
What fits with you about using the medicine and what doesn't?
Did you want to continue with it?

---

Next, asking Alexis her opinion about the methylphenidate authorized her as the expert on her experience of the medicine. As in other kinds of re-authoring conversations, I then asked questions to flesh out and enrich her description of her experience:

S: What's been positive?
ALEXIS: When I took the bus before, if it was crowded, it would be too hard for me to stay on it, but now I can think clear and process

enough to realize that I'm okay. Like the other day, I lost my food stamp card and I was able on my own to take the bus over to the office and get a new card and return home. What felt good was for once in my life I ran into a problem and could take care of it myself.

S: (Writing notes.) It felt good to be able to take care of the problem yourself. And why is that important to you?

Alexis: This is important to me because although I'm doing pretty good in general, I am not at my potential of what I am capable of. I'm planning on starting college and I will need to be able to overcome problems to do that. I want to go into psychology and be a therapist, and I want to get focused enough to not make everything a crisis, and not run for cover whenever there is a problem.

S: Do I have this right? (reading back from notes) With the Ritalin, you can process enough when you are on the bus to know that you are okay. Your thinking is clear enough to let you do new things on your own, like replace a lost food stamp card, which involved taking a bus to a new place, speaking with the office people, and taking the bus back home. It felt great to find out that you can take care of a problem by yourself, and this is important to you because you will be facing problems when you get to college that you will need to take care of. You know you are not yet at your potential. You are planning to study psychology and become a therapist, and to do that you want to be focused enough to deal with the problems that come up without making them a crisis or needing to run for cover.

After generating a fuller description of Alexis's experience of using methylphenidate, I asked the kind of *why* question that invites further development of the story of Alexis's dreams and commitments, and then retold the story to strengthen and rehearse it. Strengthening the story of Alexis's values and commitments was intended to enhance how she experienced herself and her life. She had newly discovered and articulated the story of her ability and desire to take care of her own problems and become a therapist who could help other people take care of theirs, and this story was now available to her as a powerful resource. Furthermore, developing the conversation in this way implicitly placed the medicine in the position of serving Alexis's vision. Our conversation continued:

S: So is the Ritalin doing what you had hoped it would?

ALEXIS: Yup. I think the Ritalin is helping. If you agree, can I higher it up?

S: Let me ask you a few questions first. Any negative effects?

ALEXIS: Like what?

S: Shakiness?

ALEXIS: No.

S: Pounding heart?

ALEXIS: No.

S: Sleeping okay?

ALEXIS: I never sleep well, but my sleep is the same as always.

S: How about appetite and eating?

ALEXIS: I've noticed that I feel hungry more often.

S: You do? That's not usual with Ritalin. If you want to increase the Ritalin a little, it would be safe to try it.

ALEXIS: I do.

You can hear how repeatedly asking Alexis's opinion of the methylphenidate and its effects authorized her as the expert. She decided whether the Ritalin was helpful, whether to continue it, and whether to increase the dose. In this part of the conversation, after briefly getting Alexis's opinion about the higher dose of Ritalin, I asked about the kinds of negative effects for which Ritalin is known. Here, I was the expert on the medicine, and Alexis was the expert on her experience of the medicine. Soliciting the story of potential negative effects of a medicine creates space to allow a story to emerge of how the medicine might not be serving the person's needs. It is not unlike exploring the possible negative aspects of any story or practice. Offering specific questions can make it easier for someone to reveal a problem that they might not wish to trouble their doctor or therapist about. I was reasonably reassured that methylphenidate was not causing Alexis problems and I offered Alexis information about the medicine and a prescription for a higher dose as she preferred.

I next met with Alexis one month later.

S:  What has it been like taking the higher dose of Ritalin?

ALEXIS:  It's more helpful. I noticed that I'm able to deal with situations I usually wouldn't be able to deal with.

S:  Like what?

ALEXIS:  I hate hospitals, I hate 'em, I can't stand 'em, but my aunt went to surgery and I went everyday to see her, sometimes until 11 p.m. I'd take the bus over and over to get there. I would not be able to take the bus without Ritalin.

S:  What about taking Ritalin makes it more possible to take the bus?

ALEXIS:  The Ritalin does not get me over my fear or anything. With it, I can say to myself, *OK, I'm unfamiliar with this bus, but I know it will get me where I want to go, even if I have to transfer.* It gives me enough ground to understand, to know what I am doing. And to know that even if I end up at the wrong destination, it's no biggy.

S:  With Ritalin, you can think it through?

ALEXIS:  Yes. Before the Ritalin, even taking the bus every day, I would ask myself, *Am I doing it right?* With Ritalin, I know I'm okay, I know what I'm doing. Even if I don't do it right, I have enough time to spare. I can laugh when I make a mistake, instead of being like *Oh my god!*

S:  (Pause.)

ALEXIS:  I don't know if it's the Ritalin. I have to say it's partially the Ritalin. I can laugh at my own experience—I always could—now I can laugh at more situations. I'm no longer feeling like if I make a mistake I'm ruining everyone's life or screwing up the progress.

Here we were again considering the effects of the medicine, with Alexis as the expert. As she was talking about the benefits she was attributing to the methylphenidate, I was thinking of how to invite forward the story of how it was Alexis's agency and commitments that made it possible for her to visit her aunt in the hospital. My intention was to be sure that Alexis was not attributing her accomplishments to the medicine instead of to herself. Mis- or overattribution of preferred developments to medicine is common unless it is explicitly countered. Medicines are never the reason why someone is able to take successful action. Such success is due to the person's talents, abilities, commitments, and vision. The medicine may be making those abilities and intentions more available to the person, but medicine does not impart the ability to do algebra, the vision to get a GED, the value of visiting relatives in the hospital, or the talent of having a sense of humor. The story that positive developments are *due to* medicine curtails opportunities for preferred identity development, while the story that positive things are due to the person's intentions and agency, which might be more available to them because of medicine, creates opportunities for preferred identity development.

In my pause in this dialogue, I was searching for a helpful question to create just such opportunities. But I didn't have to ask anything—Alexis herself set the medicine in perspective and honored her own skills and values. The story of Alexis's ability to laugh at situations offered possibilities for more richly tracing the history of Alexis's skills, values, and knowledge about her life, possibilities which I took up in a meeting with her several months later. Alexis succeeded in reaching her goal of getting a paid job, and she was working as a salesperson at a discount department store as she continued to participate in an educational program to help her get her GED. She came in saying she was exhausted from her long work week and described her difficulties with her manager.

ALEXIS: The first weeks I took it personal, then I noticed he has this personality where he wants everyone to know he has authority and can boss everyone around. So now I can laugh when he bitches at me.

S: Being able to laugh like that, is that a skill you've used before?

ALEXIS: I've had to use it all my life. Since I was a little kid, other kids made fun of me and beat me up because of my tremor.

S: What helped you get through that?

ALEXIS: Katrina, my stepsister. She had mental retardation and got beat up worse than me. She was a lot younger but we went to the same school. I had to be her strength. I had to be tough so she wouldn't see me break down. No matter what happened to me, it didn't hurt as much as seeing her get made fun of. I laid down the law with the other kids. I was her protector.

S: What difference did it make to her that you stepped in, in that way?

ALEXIS: A really big difference. She felt close to me.

S: What does it mean to you to have been helpful to Katrina?

ALEXIS: It means a lot, because she was so important in my life.

S: Being helpful to someone like you were to Katrina, is that linked to hopes and dreams you have now?

ALEXIS: Yes, my hopes to get my GED and start college in September and maybe get to be a therapist myself. So many people have helped me get where I am today. It'll be hard to leave the program [helping her prepare for the GED], they've all been there for me.

S: What do you think it means to them that you are taking this next step?

ALEXIS: They are proud of how much they have helped me, but just like you and your obnoxiousness (shared laughter), they're not taking credit, they say it's me, that I did it. I did something, of course. I reached out my hand and all you guys dragged me out of the mud and dirt to get me where I am today.

S: What made it possible for you to reach out like that?

ALEXIS: Before Westfield, I had no one. I was drugged up, in bed all the time. I OD'd nine times. I raised hell, called crisis every night. I blamed them because they weren't willing to reach out. They couldn't stand me because I couldn't stand me. Finally, after my therapist Becky and other people were caring to me, I learned to be caring to me, too.

As is often my experience, in this conversation with Alexis openings for preferred story development were bountiful, and it was a delight to explore a few of them with her. This was not the end of Alexis's story, but here I stop for now. She and I continued to meet for several more years, engaging in re-authoring conversations, evaluating medicines, and simply enjoying each other's company. She did indeed get her GED, and several years later, had a daughter, whom I had the pleasure of meeting. When she brought her to my office, I could see Alexis parenting her daughter with love and care.

Alexis read an earlier draft of this chapter and offered suggestions for telling her story in a way she felt was most in tune with her values. Her main suggestion, which I have made, was to resist "sugarcoating" her story, but rather to include how severe her problems had been, including repeatedly leading her to attempt to take her life. She also offered a poem to be included, part of which goes as follows:

> Who I Wish I Could Be
> By Alexis Gray
> Okay, I'll tell you but you can't laugh,
> It's someone I met years ago,
> She was someone who gave me strength to believe.
> She hasn't aged much but I love when she's around.
> Don't tell her I said this but I think she's a weirdo,
> However she does know how to follow her dreams:
> The person I wish I could be is me.
> I just want to believe and follow my dreams,
> I just want to show the best part of me.

## NARRATIVE PSYCHOPHARMACOLOGY IN SUMMARY

I have found my efforts to practice narrative psychopharmacology to be useful to the people who consult with me and gratifying for me to develop and practice. Key aspects of narrative psychiatry with regard to psychopharmacology include:

- Helping a person develop a statement of position on the problem lets them become more in touch with and energized by the story of their preferred identity, and also clarifies whether they find it useful to think of the problem as having biological components that could be constrained by medication.

- Obtaining a history of resistance to a problem clarifies and strengthens the person's knowledge and skills in resisting the problem. If medicine has been part of their resistance, they can evaluate to what extent the medicine has or has not been helpful. In this, they can compare the effects of the medicine with their own intentions and preferences. In doing so, re-authoring in the service of preferred identity development is combined with evaluation of the medicine.

- The knowledge and practices of psychopharmacology are composed of stories that can be deconstructed and examined to reveal their underlying values. Awareness of the different stories that are influencing us helps us to comply with the patient's values and preferences in making medication recommendations.

- The person's experience of a medicine depends on the medicine's biological effects and on the meanings the person ascribes to the effects. The meanings attributed to biological effects depend on the person's preferences and values, which can be elicited and strengthened through re-authoring conversations in ways that allow the person to experience her life more as she prefers.

Narrative psychopharmacologic consultations are often complex in that a variety of important yet contradictory discourses need to be considered. At the same time, bringing forward fresh moments of success in resisting problems and in experiencing life in preferred ways offers narrative psychiatrists consistent opportunities to share joy and inspiration in their work with the people who consult with them.

When someone is considering using medicine, developing stories that understand that problems are unwanted and are separate from the person, and that fortitude and valor are needed to resist symptoms, has many benefits. Narrative ways of working increase compassion, energize the person in his or her work to overcome the problem, develop and strengthen resistance to symptoms, deepen and broaden aspects of life that are uninfluenced by the problem, and let medicine offer possible biological benefits unimpeded by associations of shame.

## THE ETHICS OF CARE WHEN PROBLEMS ARE LIFE THREATENING

One of our greatest challenges as providers of mental health care is when we are faced with a situation in which a patient with overwhelming suicidal urges or life-threatening psychotic symptoms does not wish to utilize psychiatric resources that could be life saving, such as hospitalization. This issue is important and complex, and addressing it thoroughly is beyond the scope of this book. However, the values and practices of narrative psychiatry can help guide us. Narrative psychiatry honors the autonomy and authority of our patients and brings forward narratives of their values, strengths, and resources, seeking to differentiate these from the intentions and effects of problems. It guides us to pay attention to issues of privilege and marginalization and to respond in ways that are culturally attuned.

What this means is that in conversations in which potentially life-threatening problems are discussed, such as suicidal urges, we can take care to come to a thorough and nuanced understanding about the exact nature of the problem and to thoroughly understand the resources and protective factors that mitigate against the risk of harm. Many people have values and resources, such as a commitment to parents or children, that constrain them from acting on even powerful suicidal urges, or communities that will care for them and keep them safe.

Second, with patients who are presenting with problems that might become life threatening or life ruining, such as bipolar disorder, we can speak proactively about how they would want to handle possible exacerbations. Not only does this orient us to a range of resources we can draw on, but it also clarifies what values the patient would most like to honor. For example, someone may be able to clarify that he wants us to hospitalize him if he become severely manic, even though when he is in that state he says he doesn't want to go.

---

**Sample Questions to Collaboratively Plan for Responding to Life-Threatening Problems**

If the mania comes back and disrupts your life, what are your preferences for how we should handle it?

What are all the things we can put on your safety plan to help you if suicidal urges come back?

Is there someone in your life that you trust to help guide you with decisions about when it might be time to go to the hospital?

If there is a recurrence of depression that brings with it suicidal urges you don't think you can resist, what are your preferences for how I should help you stay safe?

If it seems you have completely lost hope and might kill yourself and hospitalization appears to be the only way to keep you safe, which hospital would you prefer we use?

---

Third, in having these conversations, we can be transparent about our own values. For example, I am transparent about my value that I will take action that might save someone's life. This honors my patients' autonomy, in that they can choose whether or not they want to work with me or what they say to me. I have come to hold this value from my experience of having patients for whom I have authorized involuntary hospitalization for suicide risk come back and thank me for saving their lives. Others of us may hold different values for different but equally compelling reasons.

Of course there are times when someone comes into our care in a life-threatening situation with whom we not yet had a conversation about his or her preferences for handling it. We are called upon to best discern what the patient would want us to do if there were no problem constraining their reasoning, but often we cannot know what that is. In these situations we are nonetheless called upon to act, and we each shall do so in accordance with our own values.

Last, those of us who work in a psychiatric crisis service or hospital can partner with people who might use mental health services to develop therapeutic protocols that optimize respect for patients, expand therapeutic options, and minimize coercive or traumatizing practices. Although we who are psychiatrists, psychiatric nurses, psychologists, and social workers in hospital settings are often constrained by policies and financial realities over which we have little control, we can nonetheless identify the next steps we might take to help our organizations begin to move toward an ethic of care that honors our values.

Psychiatry is seeking ways to offer more sensitive, person-centered care. Mental health recovery[14] and trauma-informed care[15] initiatives are emblematic of this call for greater respect for and collaboration with patients. The strengths-based, collaborative practices of narrative psychiatry offer ways to more fully exemplify the principles of both recovery and trauma-informed care, honoring patients' experiences and preferences and partnering with them to promote wellness.

## Notes

1. http://www.activeminds.org/
2. http://www.nami.org/
3. http://www.ocfoundation.org/
4. http://www.dbsalliance.org
5. http://www.hearingvoicesusa.org/
6. http://theicarusproject.net/
7. http://www.mindfreedom.org/campaign/madpride
8. Irving Kirsch et al., "Initial Severity and Antidepressant Benefits: A Meta-Analysis of Data Submitted to the Food and Drug Administration," *PLoS Med* 5, no. 2 (2008): e45. doi:10.1371/journal.pmed.0050045; Irving Kirsch, *The Emperor's New Drugs: Exploding the Antidepressant Myth* (New York: Basic Books, 2010).
9. Whitaker, *Anatomy of an Epidemic*.
10. Chana Joffe-Walt, "Unfit for Work: The Startling Rise of Disability in America," National Public Radio, accessed April 15, 2013, http://apps.npr.org/unfit-for-work/.
11. Jaako Seikkula, "Five-Year Experience of First-Episode Nonaffective Psychosis Treated in Open-Dialogue Approach: Treatment Principles, Follow-Up Outcomes, and Two Case Studies," *Psychotherapy Research* 16 (2006): 214–28.

12. Henry Greely et. al., "Toward Responsible Use of Cognitive-Enhancing Drugs by the Healthy," *Nature* 456 (December 10, 2008): 702–5.

13. Michael White and Alice Morgan, *Narrative Therapy with Children and Their Families* (Adelaide, Australia: Dulwich Centre Publications, 2006), 71.

14. "Recovery Support," accessed January 11, 2013, Substance Abuse and Mental Health Services Administration, http://www.samhsa.gov/recovery/.

15. "Welcome to the National Center for Trauma Informed Care," accessed January 11, 2013, http://www.samhsa.gov/nctic/default.asp.

# PART TWO

# Narrative Psychiatry in Practice

# CHAPTER SEVEN

# Finding Lost Stories of Love

*Remembering Love and Legacy amid Loss*

"'I have no son Danny,'" Daniel said, with bitterness. "That's what my father said to me when he was near death. Thirteen years ago, I go to see him in the hospital, and he's there in the bed with tubes coming out of him. I go up to him and he says, 'Who's that?' and I say, 'It's your son, Danny,' and he says, 'Danny who? I have no son Danny.'" Daniel's face bore traces of sadness and anger. "Just before he died he denied me."

Daniel Francis O'Conner, a spirited man of sixty-seven, sat perched in the middle of the couch in my bright, airy private-practice office. He had the time and resources to engage in weekly, open-ended psychotherapy with me. With a short white beard, sparkling blue eyes, a quick smile that lit up his whole face, and a readiness to laugh at himself and the world, Daniel had an equal readiness to hold himself and the world to high standards of generosity, morality, and justice. I looked forward to our meetings, in which Daniel moved from one story of his life to another with eloquence, grit, irony and humor like a true *seanachaí*, an Irish storyteller.

A lifelong resident of Holyoke, a tough little city in Massachusetts known for its historic mills and factories, Daniel shared the feisty passion of its Irish-immigrant residents. He was married to his beloved wife, Molly, and they had two grown children, Brigid, age 30, and James, 25. A published poet who was newly retired from thirty-two years as an award-winning high school English teacher and long retired from boxing, Daniel was exploring a new career as a psychotherapist. He had met me at a workshop on narrative psychiatry that I had given at The Family Institute of Cambridge (the one in which I had presented my work with Elena, from chapter 5), and wanted to work with me, with hopes of taking stock of what his legacy might be as he prepared to enter his seventies.

Our meandering weekly conversations over six months offered enough pith and drama for a whole book; in this chapter I will consolidate conversations that took place over several sessions to follow themes of love and legacy as they evolved under the touch of re-authoring questions I occasionally proffered amid Daniel's thoughts and recollections. In this, we will see narrative approaches for renegotiating definitions of success and for remembering loved ones.

## ORIGINS

Daniel was born in 1939, and there were seven siblings in his family of origin, "four ghosts and three substantials." His oldest brother died in infancy, and then, during Daniel's early childhood, two younger brothers and a younger sister died at birth. "I am the youngest of the three that lived. I was three pounds and pronounced dead before I was born. So much for the mists reading the future…."

His father dropped out of school in the second grade and worked at many jobs, starting with bootlegging when he was eight years old. He went on to work in the local mills, for a program in the WPA (the federally funded Depression-era Works Progress Administration), as a bus driver, and as a bartender in a working-class pub. Later he became city councilor, senior tax examiner, and, finally, state legislator. "He was a scrapper who understood 'the streets,'" Daniel said of him.

Daniel's mother was the only member of her family of seven siblings to graduate from high school, after which she began working as a waitress and later, in a mill "with an oppressive atmosphere." Daniel said, "My mother's parents immigrated from the extreme poverty of the West of Ireland around 1900. My father's parents emigrated earlier to escape injustice and starvation—*an Gorta Mór*, the Great Hunger—in the 1850s."

During Daniel's childhood, "neither parent would admit they were Irish," insisting that they were simply "American."

When Daniel was three years old, his father and most of the other men in his extended family joined the military to fight in World War II and were stationed in Europe. His cousin Patrick died there, and Daniel remembers the gold star they had in the window in his honor. With the loss of the babies and the absence of the men, Daniel said, "the whole family became depressed. I was a sensitive kid and I took it all in." For the three years that the men were gone, from age three to six, Daniel didn't speak. "The first thing I ever saw on TV was the Nuremberg Trials and tapes of the concentration camps and bodies being bulldozed into mass graves. There was no one there to help me make sense of that. There was a lot of chaos in my family at that time. When my father and uncles came home from the war, I opened up again," he said. "Then I talked like a volcano, and," he added with a twinkle, "I haven't stopped since."

Soon after the men returned, his maternal grandfather, Daniel F. O'Driscoll, a primary figure his life, died. Upon his return from the war, his father worked three jobs to make ends meet, and Daniel felt his absence. "I remember a lot of aloneness and loneliness as a child. Sitting on the curb at age three playing with ants. There were brooks and woods near us, and I would go there—I had a relationship with nature." He went to Catholic school and had nuns for his teachers, some of whom he cherished. "Sister Clarice would hug me and I would just melt. I vowed to be the best student in the room." At home, there was virtually no physical affection.

Up to age thirteen, Daniel characterized himself as a "quiet, holy boy who wanted to be a priest." But after puberty he became increasingly wild and was always getting into brawls. "Every Irish family needs to have a screwup, and that bounced around in my family and landed on me. My mother wanted to be able to control me and she was not able to. She used to call me 'a son of a bitch.'" He began boxing, and he was good at it. He dropped out of high school. At age eighteen, he read *Finnegan's Wake*. "There was this great part in the book about a river flowing, and suddenly it hit me—everything I learned about Jesus was a myth. I felt nauseous, as if the whole world was taken out from under me. There was no one I could talk to about this. I was in the tribe but I wasn't a member." He described himself as angry and bitter and exuding a sense of rage through his adulthood, and he boxed with a vengeance. About fighting he said, "Either I win or you kill me."

## CLARIFYING LEGACY

"I feel a sense of anxiety and vulnerability," Daniel said in our first meeting, smiling wryly, "because two or three years ago I realized that I was going down the other side of the mountain." His mortality was staring him in the face and he was seeking answers to questions such as, "Who am I? What will my legacy be, especially to my wife and children? And then, to the larger community?"

Daniel could tell me the admiring comments his teachers, colleagues, students, and clients made about him, but he didn't feel a consistent sense of his own merit. He said, "In recent years, my wife, my daughter, and my son have been telling me that I have gifts, and I am wanting to let that in, but I struggle with really believing it. The story I have is that I have a deficit—from early childhood, from my family."

As we spoke, I was thinking of how I might support the new story that Daniel was cultivating about what his gifts and his legacy might be, a story that offered an alternative to a deficit-laced story of identity. Stories of deficit or failure invite us to help our patients clarify what definitions of success they value. Success and failure are not absolute categories, but are always determined in relation to particular standards. Not infrequently, our patients are laboring to meet, and evaluating themselves against, criteria for success as defined by others that do not actually fit their own most cherished values. I suspected that Daniel, in his questions about his legacy, was experiencing normalizing judgments that narrowly defined what a successful legacy might be and that missed the richness and individuality of a legacy based on his personal values. Instead, we could develop the story of what legacy he personally would want to leave; that is, what he valued most. Then I could invite him to give me examples of when he stayed true to those values and had succeeded in manifesting his gifts. In doing so, I am inspired by the work of Michael White, as exemplified in his work on deconstructing failure.[1]

---

**Sample Questions to Deconstruct Failure and to Elicit Personal Stories of Success**

When you say that you failed in that way, what was it that you failed in relation to? That is, what value were you not fully living up to?

How important to you is that particular value?

Were there other values that you were staying true to in that instance?

In terms of values that are important to you, are there other moments in your life in which someone might see a sign of your commitment to those values?

What would your own personal definition of living a successful life be?

What might someone see in your life that is evidence of living your life in that way?

Have there been times that someone else has appreciated the ways in which you have manifested your gifts?

---

One way to elicit narratives of success is to ask the patient to tell stories of times when others appreciated his gifts. Daniel told me about a colleague with a PhD from Harvard, with whom he went through a training program in executive coaching, in which they coached each other. "He really gets a boot out of me. He calls me Danger Dan, because of how I went from being a street kid and a boxer to a poet and a therapist. He loved what I was doing. I used a metaphor with him about how he was a knight in armor, but the armor was blocking his heart. He said he wanted to open the armor, but he realized that he left his heart at Harvard—and now he wanted it back. After that conversation, he wanted me to offer executive coaching for these CEOs he knew. He said, 'What the boardroom needs is you.'"

"Do these stories exemplify something that you value?" I asked.

"The corporate world is heartless," he said. "They need someone who can play hardball *and* have a big heart."

"Would that be a statement about what your legacy might be?"

"I would say my legacy is helping people put their hearts into what they do."

"Helping people put their hearts into what they do. And are there other ways in your life that you are helping people put their hearts into what they do?"

"With my kids. I wanted to give them opportunities, but even more, I wanted to teach them to open their hearts more fully." Daniel told me about how he let go of his bitterness and resentment to make more space for his children. His daughter had left her position as a stockbroker to teach high school math in a poor neighborhood in Holyoke, and his son at age 25 had created an urban gardening project, cultivating relationships with businesspeople to help fund it.

"I see that the legacy is there," Daniel said as he shared story after story, laughing. "It's just a matter of itemizing it!"

And so we went on to itemize it, clarifying Daniel's success in living out values of making connections, speaking from the heart, and promoting freedom (which he defined, in the words of Camus, as the "opportunity to do better"). Daniel valued what he called "seeing the big picture," and time and again he had stepped into complex situations with an open heart: teaching impoverished kids high school English, developing cultural centers to sustain the best of Irish values and traditions in the face of a rapidly changing world, supporting living in harmony with nature at a time of impending natural resource depletion, and using wit and humor to challenge those he felt were acting without integrity. He spoke about his value of respecting differences, reaching out to people of other cultures; caring for his friends, several of whom were dying; and promoting his value of openheartedness in professional contexts. As we continued to illuminate the brilliance of Daniel's legacy, I also invited him to consider the fact that not everyone was willing to be aware in the ways that he was or to strive to do what he did.

"You are inviting others to open their hearts in contexts in which that is uncommon," I said.

"I thought it was common," he said, modestly. "I grew up in Holyoke during the Holocaust, and now I am concerned about another apocalypse. I want to leave a legacy that is about helping people and opening their hearts. I am aging, my friends are dying. I want to learn about myself and use the potential I have for good. I want the bullshit of the former dominant story to be plowed under and to uncover a new story. I want to be able to appreciate my own brilliance."

Over the course of our conversations, the story of Daniel's legacy to his wife, his children, and the wider world was woven through with another story: his father's legacy to him.

## LOOKING FOR LOVE

"'Who the hell do you think you are?' That's what my dad would say to me, any time I tried something new or did something well," Daniel said during our first meeting together.

Daniel had worked with a psychotherapist in the 1980s, which he found very helpful. "I got in touch with my sadness and my anger at my father," he said. In the 1990s he consulted with a caring and skillful family therapist who was knowledgeable about ethnic issues, helping him understand about his Irish parents, of whom Daniel said, "If they showed any sign of weakness or affection or overt love we wouldn't stay tough—we would become vulnerable." Having an inflated sense of self was seen as harmful and dangerous. Understanding how his father's Irish heritage influenced his parenting soothed some of the bitterness and resentment Daniel felt, what he described as "the old me." He said, "I started to appreciate who I had become both despite and because of who they are."

He had become more accepting of his father's limitations, but the narrative he told about his father in our first meetings was of a man that Daniel wasn't sure loved or admired him. He told me story after story about the ways his father had responded to him in ways that were invalidating. Over several meetings, I listened carefully to what he had to say.

"He always called me a big, dumb, stupid lug," Daniel said. "He met his match with me though. He was streetwise and always helping other people, but when it came to me, there was tension. Never in my memory did he touch me or hug me or say, 'I love you.'" His father's deathbed disavowal of him, "I have no son Danny," remained a raw wound.

Daniel said that in pursuing his master's degree in psychology in his thirties, he had received top marks and glowing letters of recommendation from his supervisors. "I showed them to my father—he read them—and said, 'Too bad your brother Patrick couldn't do this.' And I thought, *Oh, you fucker.*"

"What would you have wanted to hear?" I asked.

"'Great job! Congratulations! Wow! You're amazing!'" Daniel said feelingly.

"What difference would it have made to you if he had said that?"

"I would have found a way to get a PhD at Harvard! As it was, I just put that aside and got on with life."

"And what kind of support would your father have needed to have been able to say that to you?" I asked. In this, I was drawing on the work of Sallyann Roth and Richard Chasin,[2] who developed such questions to open up new understandings of what might have been possible, had our loved ones had the support they would have needed to have been able to manifest their most loving intentions. These "mythic stories" in "imaginary time" offer our patients a chance to feel love that might have been obscured.

### Sample Questions to Enhance Compassion and Discover a Story of Loving Intentions

At that time of difficulty/joy, what would you have wanted from your mother?

What difference would it have made to you if you had had that response from her?

What kind of support would your mother have needed, then and in her earlier life, to have been able to give you what you needed then?

What difference would it have made to her life and to your life, if she had had that support?

Daniel sat back on the couch and looked at me, pausing as he appeared to search for words. "My father? What would *he* have needed?" Daniel clenched and unclenched his jaw, looked away, then right back at me. "He needed love. He needed someone to say to him, 'You're quite the guy.' I remember talking with him once on the phone. He was outgoing, gregarious even. He was sixty-two then. He had so much more to contribute than he'd had a chance to. I said, 'I love you, Dad.' He couldn't take it in." Daniel paused, thinking back. "My dad's father was passive and his mother, my grandmother, was cruel. His sister Edith died of cancer. His brother Sean burnt to death in a fire after the two of them went through the war together. My father then raised Sean's daughter. He took care of all of us. He could have rages at home, but he was a generous guy, altruistic to a fault. He was funny, witty, he told stories. He and I, we connected every so often...." Daniel smiled. "It's no wonder that I became a boxer. My dad got in a fistfight once in a meeting when somebody insulted someone in the family."

Daniel's father taught him to fight. "When Billy Gallagher punched me in the nose, I went home and told my dad and he said, 'Punch him back.' One year later, Billy hit me again, so after school I pulverized him." Daniel smiled and raised his eyebrows. "Word got out." It seemed Daniel had what it took to be a boxer. As a young teen, he began competing in matches, and time after time, he won.

"And your father, did he come to any of your boxing matches?" I asked.

"He was always there," Daniel said.

"He was always there," I repeated. "Watching the match?"

"He was in my corner."

Amid the stories of how his father didn't care and had insulted and denied him were flickers of how his father might have acted toward Daniel in a way that could be considered loving or admiring or generous, but there was no theme, no plot that tied these alternative events into a story. They were outside of the dominant narrative and as such didn't contribute much to Daniel's sense of his father or of his father's love and admiration for him. The narrative that Daniel had developed in his initial psychotherapy was that he felt understandable sadness and anger about his father. He had begun to supplement this story with one in which his father's failings, rather than being blameworthy, were a result of his life experiences and cultural expectations and customs. The dominant story was that his father had failed to love him well. What was lost was the story of how his father had *also* succeeded in loving him well—a story I saw consistent glimmers of amid the joys, tragedies, and rambunctious exploits of Daniel's life.

What difference might it make to Daniel if the lost story of his father's love was found? That was the question on my mind as I spoke with him.

"He was in your corner?" I repeated. "Literally in your corner of the ring?" Daniel nodded.

"What did it mean to you that he was in your corner?"

Daniel paused and looked down at his hands, then back up at me. "Once my dad put a hundred-dollar bet on me to win. When I was fifteen, he signed me up for the Silver Gloves Championship. I won my division and was named the most outstanding boxer of the tournament. My dad won a hundred dollars."

"Your father bet one hundred dollars that you would win," I said.

Daniel nodded. "Seven or eight years ago, I was back in the club where the fight had been, having a drink, and I ran into Tommy, whom I used to box with. He said, 'Your father used to brag about you all the time. He called you *the champ*.'"

"Your dad bragged about you to other people. He called you *the champ*."

"To other people, maybe. To me he would just say, 'Who the hell do you think you are?'"

"He wasn't able to—or didn't choose to—compliment you to your face."

"No."

"What does it say about how your father felt about you that he bragged about you to other people?"

Daniel looked down and then back up at me with tears in his eyes. "I guess my father did appreciate and value me."

"Are there any other examples of how your father appreciated and valued you?" I asked.

"When we were buying our house, Molly and I had no money. We needed the down payment. Molly said, 'I can't ask my father.' So I said I would ask my father for the money. I was amazed, because I called him up and asked if he could loan me ten thousand dollars for the down payment. He didn't say anything, just 'Meet me at the bank.' So I go meet him out front. He says, 'Let's go in.' I said, 'What will Mom say?' He says, 'Don't worry about that.' He takes out ten thousand dollars and gives it to me."

"So your father lent you ten thousand dollars, no questions asked," I said. "What did that mean to you?"

"That was big," Daniel said. "But the next day he was back to, 'Who the hell do you think you are?'"

"I wonder what he meant when he said that."

"What do you mean?" Daniel asked.

"He would say that when you did something well, like got a good letter of recommendation, or when you wanted to try something new?"

"Yeah."

"So he noticed?"

"What?"

"Noticed that you did something well?"

Daniel smiled. "Yeah."

"I wonder if that was his way of communicating that he noticed, that you were doing something well? Saying, 'Who the hell do you think you are?'"

"I was doing things he never had the chance to do. Going to college. Getting a master's degree."

"Things that he admired, or didn't admire?"

"Things that he admired," Daniel said.

"What if when he said, 'Who the hell do you think you are?' he was expressing his admiration for you? In a particularly Irish kind of way?"

Daniel held his left fist in his right hand and gazed at me with bright, moist eyes, slowly nodding.

Our time was almost up, and there were so many questions I still wanted to ask, questions to further flesh out this nascent story, clearly moving to Daniel, about how his father admired and valued him.

"Sometimes," I said, "People welcome it if I write them a letter about our conversations together. Would that be something of interest to you?"

"Sure!"

## THERAPEUTIC LETTERS

At this point in our work, after our first eight meetings, Daniel was beginning to articulate new narratives about his father and about his legacy. New narratives are vulnerable to becoming overshadowed by previously dominant stories and disappearing. Among the many ways to strengthen a new narrative is writing therapeutic letters or creating other therapeutic documents. Therapeutic documents offer a chance to both repeat the new narratives that are emerging, preferably in the patient's own words, and to pose questions that will develop them further, questions just like you might ask in person. Most commonly, I will ask patients if they would like me to write out what they said to take with them, and right there in the session, I will transcribe onto a card or piece of paper a compelling statement they made or offer questions to take home. (I describe an example of this in my work with Elena in chapter 5.) Creating therapeutic documents within a session fits the time demands of most of our work lives. We can also create more comprehensive documents outside of sessions.

Most patients welcome receiving a letter, but of course one should always ask first. Letters are time consuming to write and are generally not billable, but are almost invariably described by patients as enormously valuable, equal in worth to multiple sessions of psychotherapy. One way I have created space in my day to write letters is to create a document that is simultaneously a letter to a patient and medical record documentation, such as a progress note or treatment summary. (An example of this is the letter I wrote to Amanda in chapter 3.) I sometimes write letters over the course of several days, using unexpected open time in my schedule when there is a cancelation or no-show.

Here is the letter I sent Daniel, edited for brevity:

April 9, 2007

Dear Daniel:

Hello, and I hope you are well. I am writing you this letter to offer a summary of our conversations.

You described your intentions for our conversations were to help you clarify your legacy to your wife Molly; to your children James and Brigid; and to the world at large. My understanding of your hope is that you wish to be able to appreciate your own gifts and to illuminate your own brilliance. Understanding your own legacy is especially compelling to you at this time of life, as you are experiencing the deaths of your contemporaries and anticipating your own mortality.

As you begin understanding what your legacy might be, you have identified things that are essential to you. One is helping people bring their hearts into what they do and open their hearts more fully. You yourself have brought your openheartedness more and more fully into your relationships with Molly and your children, letting go of bitterness and resentment so that you could be more present and caring with them. In addition you have told many stories of your success in helping bring your clients' hearts into what they do, and have been increasingly recognized for your gifts in this area. Other aspects of your legacy and the values and skills that you hold include being able to see the big picture and recognizing painful truths. You also value learning, humor, boldness, and poetry. You have written hundreds of poems and have been recognized for your skill.

As you examine your own legacy, it brings forward stories of your father's legacy to you. We have been discussing some of the evidence of your father's love and admiration for you across cultures and generations that divide you. You have described evidence of his love, including him lending you $10,000 without question to put a down payment on your house, his standing in your corner both literally and metaphorically when you have been fighting, and we are questioning whether his question to you of "Who the hell do you think you are?" may be a sign of both his admiration for you and all that you have become as well as his love for you manifest in his desire to do right by you as a father and prevent you from the harm that can befall someone with an inflated view of themselves. Evidence of his admiration includes the way he bragged about you frequently at work and the $100 bet he put on you because he was confident that you could fight. I am curious about other ways that your father showed his love for you and for others and other ways that his admiration for you can be detected in his life.

Daniel, there are so many directions questions could go in from these topics of conversation about which we have been speaking. For example: What did it mean to your father that you wanted and let him be in your corner? What if every time your father said, "Who the hell do you think you are?" he meant, "You are amazing and I want you to thrive?"

Other questions are: What is it that motivated you and allowed you to let go of bitterness and resentment? In what ways were they not serving you? What does your wife Molly most appreciate about you? What words or phrases that you have used with her will stay with her forever?

And finally: What gift is it to your children for you to understand your own brilliance?

Please consider this letter part of an ongoing conversation and by no means any definitive statement. It would be impossible to capture the poetic richness of our conversations in a letter as brief as this one. I look forward to your response at our next meeting.

Fondly,

SuEllen Hamkins, M.D.

## FINDING LOST STORIES OF LOVE

Narrative psychiatry looks for lost stories of love, love that was present in our patients' lives but was not part of their story of who they are. In doing so, it draws inspiration from the "re-membering practices" developed by

White, introduced originally in his 1988 paper entitled, "Saying Hullo Again: The Incorporation of the Lost Relationship in the Resolution of Grief."[3] Remembering practices are intended to identify people, living or dead, who have made an important contribution to a person's life and then to flesh out and vivify the story of mutual positive influence. In doing so, White emphasizes that in addition to tracing the contribution of the valued person to the patient's life, we can further develop cherished aspects of our patients' identities by inviting them to describe how the valued person might have seen them and to articulate what contributions the patient made to the valued person's life and identity.[4]

In our conversation and in the letter I sent him, I asked Daniel questions to find lost stories of his father's love. My intention in this was not to deny but rather to supplement Daniel's experience of his father's limitations with the missing story of his father's skills and intentions in loving.

### Sample Questions to Find Lost Stories of Love

What did your grandmother do that you found helpful to you?

Did your father show up for you in any way?

What did it mean to you that your dad was there for you in that way?

If you could imagine how your mother might describe you, what might she say?

Did you take in the kindness that your neighbor offered to you, or did you reject it?

How might your friend's life have been enhanced by your willingness to share what was so important to them?

What might it mean to your cousin that you welcomed her support?

If that author could know how their book influenced your life, what difference might that make to that author's sense of self?

## CULTIVATING STORIES OF LOVE AND LEGACY

"I showed Molly the letter you sent me," Daniel said, his eyes crinkling as he smiled. "She saw that question about what she most appreciates about me and answered it." He paused, his face filled with emotion. "What was most moving to me of what she said was, 'You've been the mother I never had.' Molly got nothing from her own mother. The more Molly tried to get affection from her mother, the more her mother resented it."

"When Molly said, 'You've been the mother I never had,' what was she referring to?" I asked.

"The more she tried to get affection from me, the more affection I gave her," Daniel said, smiling. "She said that what I gave her was so essential to who she is. With me she was able to open up to her own cre-ativity. We share artistic values. She was able to appreciate her gifts as a musician playing the violin, as a painter, as an artist, with drawing, dance, and design. She's an amazing person." Daniel paused, his eyes welling up. "She asked me what did *I* get from our relationship. And the look in her face—so beautiful—such loveliness. I said, 'You point out things that I don't see. You take me to these beautiful places.'" Tears were falling from Daniel's eyes, and my own eyes were welling up. He smiled and gestured toward his face. "Here I go again."

"Is that okay with you?" I asked gently.

"It's not the usual thing for a boxer from Holyoke," he joked.

I paused, staying present, feeling our emotional connection, gazing warmly at Daniel but saying nothing, aware of both how moved he was and of his discomfort with shedding tears, wanting to give him the space to feel what he was feeling and then to choose what direction our con-versation moved in.

Daniel wiped off the tears. "For both of us, we listen and acknowledge one another. That means so much." Then he smiled mischievously. "Molly gets a boot out of me. She said, 'I never had so much fun as being married to you. I never know what's going to happen.'

"And my daughter Brigid," he went on, "she had an experience of her own with 'Who the hell do you think you are?' She told me she was talking with some colleagues about starting a charter school with a social justice theme, and they said something half-admiring, half-insulting, which led her to think maybe she shouldn't. It was just as if they had said, 'Who the hell do you think you are?' and I thought, *We don't get it about our own brilliance.* Brigid said, 'I have to get more experience first,' and I asked her, 'How will you know when you're ready?' and she said, 'I'm probably there now.' And I said, 'Listen to yourself.'

"And James. He is going to open a worker-owned restaurant in Holyoke." Daniel beamed. "James is grounded in his values of who we are as human beings in relation to everything. He respects the dignity of everyone."

Daniel looked me in the eye. "What you wrote in that letter, it made me see how my father showed his love—to me and to others. All these stories came flooding back." Daniel spoke of his father's legacy, how he saw the burden on the poor people of Holyoke and took action to help them, as a citizen and in his role as city councilor and state senator. He saw ways in which his father valued and appreciated him, such as bringing him along to help him connect with people when he was campaigning. "He had an appreciation of me. He saw me do things. He noticed the work I did to repair the house. He couldn't help me with my homework, but he noticed that I was one of the best students at school. He appreciated my abilities as a boxer. He saw that I could do the work of three men. He got me several jobs. He said to me, 'All I ask is that you work your ass off.'

"Whatever he attended to, I attended to. When I graduated from trade school, the contractor I was working for kept me on, but at the same rate. My father told me to ask my boss for a raise. I know my father must have spoken to him, because he gave me the raise and also bought me a new suit! Then a better, less grueling job opened up, and my father wanted me to have that job. He fought like hell to get me that job, with benefits and paid vacation." Daniel smiled and looked at me levelly. "I got the job."

"Would that be an example of how your father was in your corner?" I asked.

"Yes, absolutely."

"What difference did it make to you that your father was in your corner?"

Daniel paused, tears again arising. "The fact that my father was in my corner," he said, "that's *why* I was a champion." We sat quietly together for a moment, taking in that realization.

"James, he's going to open the restaurant on my sixty-eighth birthday," Daniel went on. "Right near the high school where I taught for eighteen years. It's really hitting home. The impact that I have had on them. James has just turned twenty-five, and he is taking this risk. And why he's taking it: to be of service. I've been going around with him door to door, inviting families to participate."

"What your son and daughter are doing," I asked, "what does that say about you as a parent?"

Daniel smiled. "I must be doing something right. We have this unique bond. There is a huge part of me in them. And a huge part of my father in them. Like my dad was in my corner, I want to be in their corner."

"Your father's legacy to you, your legacy to your children."

"When I look around at my friends and colleagues, seeing their so-called 'success' and what their legacy will be, and I look at my life and legacy, it's clear. I would rather have what I have."

"What is it that you have, that you would rather have?" I asked.

"The legacy I want to leave my children. Clear minds, tied to their values. Big hearts. Having fun and a sense of humor." He sighed and shook his head. "It seems so simple. I am celebrating my kids. With them, there is always laughter and humor." His eyes crinkled up with a smile. "Sometimes biting humor." Daniel laughed. "I really get a boot out of myself."

At our last session, after six months of working together, I asked Daniel to reflect on his journey. "I had made up a story, that because of all the tragedies, I would die with a deficit. But now, I see that I really am different. When I let in who I am and fully appreciate that, I realize, first of all," with a tilt of his head, "*don't get grandiose,* and then," with seriousness, "*you can have a huge impact, just by being who you are.*"

His magnificent smile lit up his face. "Goethe said, 'Whatever you dream you can do, begin it. Boldness has genius, power and magic in it.'" He gazed at me with satisfaction. "I'm bold. What do I want to do? Write a poem? Write a memoir? Or take the energy left to me on this planet in another direction?"

As we prepared to say goodbye, Daniel looked at me warmly. "This has been a jaunty stroll into who I am. The gait of my soul is more bouncy now. Thank you. I appreciate that. And *Molly* appreciates that." His blue eyes sparkled. "I feel that by the time I am ninety, I will be able to say *I am who I want to be.*"

## DANIEL'S REFLECTION

Five years later, after reading this chapter, Daniel offered the following reflection:

Repeatedly, I had pressed a searing iron over the moth-eaten fabric of my life. The holes in this tattered cloth caused unease and shredded parts of me. I had a history of feeling "not being enough" and of struggling with the meaning and purpose in my life. "Who the hell do you think you are," "you big dumb lug"—these phrases I heard from my father as a kid were snares in pieces of me. They overwhelmed me and caused what I felt were irreparable wounds. I was riddled with bitterness and doubt.

It was fortuitous that Dr. SuEllen Hamkins and I met at a Narrative Therapy workshop. SuEllen provided a safe context for meaningful conversations and for my dominant narrative to change, for the affectionate threads to knit together. I have never had such a shabby and ragged relationship with anyone as I had with 'my old man'. In our work together, SuEllen helped me "thicken" stories that did not support or sustain my problem-laden, threadbare story. She helped me to see, taste, hear, smell, and touch images that sparked my imagination. I rubbed shoulders with new strands of myself, and our work uncovered and then wove "richly described" relationships between my deceased father and me.

From a non-judgmental and inquisitive stance, she listened to and recorded in detail what I shared with her. My bitterness around my relationship with my father was a heavy shawl that was, bit by bit, fashioned into love. I began to appreciate and honor my father's abundant gifts to me and to realize that our relationship was, in my evolving story, filled with loving intentions. I stopped turning against my 'old man' and turned toward him. Over time, my experience of my relationship with my father mended and became warm and gentle, clear and richly embroidered.

A letter SuEllen wrote and sent to me contained thought-provoking questions and had a meaningful and inspiring impact on our work together. The letter still provides the opportunity to reflect on long forgotten pieces of our relationship. It also reminds me of unique influences I have had on my father, my wife, my children, students, former supervisors, colleagues, and people I've worked with from around the world. This letter is a significant ally in my galaxy of allies.

With SuEllen's use of Narrative Therapy and with her abundant compassion, I learned that we are a plurality of untapped voices. We can step into new possibilities with the past and create new meanings for the future. SuEllen and I accomplished this in my relationship with my father and, paradoxically, he is more alive in my life today than he has ever been. No other therapist I had worked with had this effect on my relationship with my father, and it made room for my joyfully sauntering into relationships I had not dreamt possible.

## Notes

1. Michael White, "Addressing Personal Failure," *The International Journal of Narrative Therapy and Community Work* 3 (2002), 33–76.
2. Sallyann Roth and Richard Chasin, "Entering One Another's Worlds of Meaning and Imagination: Dramatic Enactment and Narrative Couple Therapy," in *Constructive Therapies*, ed. Michael Hoyt (New York: Guilford Publications, 1994), 189.
3. Michael White, "Saying Hullo Again: The Incorporation of the Lost Relationship in the Resolution of Grief," *Dulwich Centre Newsletter* (1988), 7–11.
4. White, *Maps,* 140.

# CHAPTER EIGHT

# Finding One's Voice

*Recovering from Trauma*

Vivian Owusu, a stunning twenty-one-year-old African woman who grew up in Ghana, was about to walk out of the university counseling center when I went to the waiting room to get her for our initial appointment. Her first psychiatric provider had retired a year after meeting her and her next one took a different job six months later, so I was her third psychiatrist in less than a year. Vivian had not shown for her first two appointments with me and now, due to a double-booking error that was my fault, I was thirty minutes late. I apologized and asked if she had time to stay and meet with me. I could see her anger and agitation. "I suppose." Irritated but still poised, Vivian followed me down the hall to my office. *What an unfortunate beginning,* I thought, feeling harried. We had been short-staffed for months and I had been squeezing patients in as best I could, feeling like I wasn't doing my best work.

Vivian settled herself upright on my couch and looked at me coolly. She had big dark eyes, flawless brown skin, beautifully braided hair, a button nose, and a hostile expression. In response to my questions, she told me she was a junior, pre-law. She hadn't slept for three or four days. Depression had been plaguing her and she had been having thoughts of killing herself. Her expression of hostility briefly showed a trace of sadness. "I don't trust people," she said. "I take things personally and I get annoyed." She often felt emotionally volatile and easily got upset with people if she felt they were rejecting her.

I had skimmed her medical record prior to the appointment and saw that she had had multiple emergency contacts with our clinicians and two psychiatric hospitalizations, the second five months earlier. She said she wasn't having suicidal thoughts currently and would call us if she did. What she wanted from me was a refill of medicines she was taking to help with the depression and anxiety. We discussed the pros and cons of the medicines, and Vivian was clear she wanted to continue with them. She was becoming slightly less irritable.

I asked her how college was for her. She liked it overall, but hadn't done as well as she had hoped the last year. She had a lot of friends and had no problem getting dates. When I asked how things were for her culturally, she said she had been in the United States since she was eleven, and it wasn't an issue. At her job as a waitress, she said it was sometimes awkward, since she was more educated than the other women of color who worked there.

## CONNECTING IN THE FACE OF TRAUMA

Halfway through that first appointment, Vivian looked at me discerningly. "I think I am having PTSD," she said.

"Would you like to say anything more about that?" I asked.

She told me the story of how she grew up in Ghana. When she was five years old her parents immigrated to the United States and left her behind with relatives, who moved her from house to house. Vivian remembered this as a very difficult time and believed she had traumatic experiences then, possibly a rape. At eleven she moved to the United States and lived variously with her older teenage sisters and family friends. Her parents divorced. Her mother was working as a live-in domestic worker and didn't have room for her, and her father became violent toward her when she tried living with him. Vivian felt that neither her parents nor her sisters were there for her then or now, and she characterized her relationships with all of them as difficult.

"Who in your family would you say you feel closest to?" I asked.

"My grandmother in Ghana. She is the one who mainly raised me. She is old now, and I hardly ever get to talk to her."

"What does your grandmother appreciate about you?"

Vivian looked slightly embarrassed, but pleased. "I don't know. I guess she sees something in me."

"What might she see in you?"

"Ummm, well, she appreciates that I am a hard worker and that I'm a 'good girl,' in her eyes. And she would be very happy and proud of what I have accomplished educationally, being in college." Vivian lowered her head and smiled shyly, raising her eyes to look up into mine.

Our time was almost up. I was grateful that it seemed that we had made it through the challenging start to the appointment and made a bit of a connection. We made a plan to meet again in two weeks. In the meantime, she would meet with her new therapist at our center. She said she felt her previous therapist didn't really care about her, because she never called her if Vivian missed an appointment.

Vivian didn't show for her next two meetings with me, nor with her therapist, but walked into the clinic the day after a missed appointment in a state of emergency, saying she was very upset and had suicidal thoughts. She had been thinking about the possibility of having been raped as a child and about her abortion last year, and in this context she had texted her ex-boyfriend, Anthony, the one who got her pregnant, but he didn't respond. So, against her better judgment she logged into his Facebook account and found out that he was in a new relationship and had changed his phone number, which upset her further. She said she felt much better after talking with the on-call clinician and rescheduled with me and with her therapist, but then didn't come to either of those appointments.

Vivian was experiencing chronic suicidal urges and traumatic memories, but wasn't coming to her appointments! I was worried and frustrated, and while I wasn't sure what would be most helpful for Vivian, I knew what would be most helpful for me: discussing the situation with colleagues who shared my values.

I have found having a peer consultation team to be an essential resource for getting support and staying true to my intentions as a practitioner, which was aptly demonstrated to me when I spoke with my team about Vivian. I have found it helpful to follow a narrative peer-supervision structure that simultaneously offers respect for the patient and support for the therapist. In one such structure,[1] the therapist wanting support is first interviewed by one member of the team for twenty to thirty minutes, while the other team members just listen. The first question to the therapist is always some variation of *What would be different if this conversation had been helpful to you?* The questions that follow invite reflection on what was going well in the treatment and what was challenging, how the therapist had overcome similar challenges in the past, how she was staying true to her values, and how she might bring those values forward more fully in the work. Then, after being interviewed, the therapist sits back and listens for about fifteen minutes as each team member shares his or her thoughts apropos what kind of input the therapist was seeking, speaking about the therapist in the third person, which gives her the luxury of just sitting back and listening. Last, the clinician shares her responses to the responses of her colleagues, followed by open conversation. We have found this structure to be useful to us as clinicians, orienting us to our values and skills, and respectful to patients.

My preference for speaking about any patient at any time is to do so in a way that is respectful and focuses on strengths as well as challenges. The stories we tell about our patients influence how we think about them and what options we develop for helping them. If we speak about patients disrespectfully or solely in pathologizing terms, we cannot help but be influenced and constrained by those narratives. Not only are disrespectful practices harmful to our patients, I believe they also undermine the point of peer supervision, which is to benefit the clinician, because such practices, even if they are intended as a joke or an opportunity to "vent," ultimately serve to decrease hope and promote burnout. One guide I use is to describe patients in ways that we would feel comfortable with them hearing.

So when it was my turn to be interviewed, I chose my work with Vivian to be the focus. "If this conversation were helpful to me, I would feel less

**One Option for Narrative Peer Supervision**

20–30 minutes
The therapist is interviewed about a patient by a colleague, while other colleagues listen.

First question: *What would be different if this conversation had been helpful to you?*

Subsequent questions elicit the story of what is going well in the treatment, what is challenging, what values the therapist is staying true to, and how the therapist might bring those values forward more fully in the work.

10–20 minutes
The therapist listens as colleagues offer their reflections on what was said, apropos the first interview question, speaking about the therapist in the third person.

5 minutes
The therapist offers his or her reflections on the reflections.

5–10 minutes
Open conversation.

worried, I would know how to get Vivian to come in and see me, and I would have a clear treatment plan." I introduced Vivian's hopes and interests, then spent the bulk of my interview speaking about my worries about her constant talk of suicide and my frustration that she only seemed to come in on-call and never when scheduled, rather self-righteously asserting that Vivian was a competent adult and it was her responsibility to keep appointments that she made, and I had a lot of other patients who could have used those time slots. When it was time to sit back and listen, I was particularly struck by what one colleague said, which was more or less, "I noticed that SuEllen said that Vivian said that she felt that her previous therapist didn't care, because she didn't call when Vivian missed her appointments. I know that SuEllen does care about Vivian, and I am wondering if Vivian could best experience that caring if SuEllen called her more than just once when Vivian doesn't come in." In the context of the roulette wheel of different psychiatrists she had been passed among, the absence of reliable family supports, and newly emerging traumatic memories, Vivian had given me a perfectly clear message about what she needed.

I called her later that day and left a message on her voicemail saying that I was thinking of her, and invited her to come in. It took less than two minutes. Calling Vivian gave her essential information about my interest and ability to be present with her. Clear boundaries with our clients is what makes our unique work possible, and what constitutes appropriate boundaries, those that are therapeutic and meet the needs of both the patient and the clinician, are different for different people. My consultation team was helpful to me in figuring out what was right for Vivian and me. Vivian didn't respond to my first call, so I called her again a few days later and left another message. The next day she called me back, crying, and said she felt she needed to be seen right away. I had an open hour and met with her immediately.

## NURTURING RECOVERY FROM TRAUMA

Vivian sat forlornly on my couch wiping tears from her eyes with the palm of her hand, holding one of my tissues in her lap. She said she was feeling sad about the abortion she had had a year earlier and described a dream in which the baby had looked at her with forgiveness. We spoke about her sadness, and I asked her what it was a testimony to. She said it was about her life, that she was suddenly aware of her life through the eyes of that unborn child. I asked what that view of her life inspired in her, and she said that it helped her to see her purpose in life, to help people. She said that she was not having suicidal thoughts, and that anyway, she couldn't kill herself because her purpose in life had not yet been fulfilled. She wanted to be happy and do more things for herself, like doing well in school, and to stop using guys to help her feel better. As she spoke, she dried her eyes and took on a look of resoluteness.

After missing her next two appointments with me, Vivian met with me six weeks later, for our third appointment. She said she was maintaining her equilibrium, using an image of the baby with whom she was briefly pregnant as a source of inspiration. She said she was coaching herself to live up to the higher standards she was setting for herself. "I'm annoyed that that boy's name, *Anthony*, keeps coming up in my mind. I don't like him and I don't miss him, so why should I want to text him? I want to act with self-respect and follow my own best advice and not get caught up in relationship drama." She noted that when she felt down, she could help herself feel better by spending time with friends, laughing, and eating good food, rather than going out to bars, drinking too much, and picking up men. Suicidal thoughts were rare and not compelling.

When I met with her a month later, she told me about her parents, neither of whom had been there for her. We spoke in detail about the familial and cultural environment in which she had grown up. As a young girl, she had had very little power. An uncle had accused her of being a "witch," which in Ghana meant she was seen as having destructive powers, and her parents had not defended her, leaving her as an unwanted pariah passed from relative to relative. Her grandmother was the only person who had taken her side. "My mother left me in a terrible situation, and now I have all this emotional baggage."

"You had to deal with a terrible situation," I said. "And somehow you did."

"It's like I was in a car accident and both my legs were broken, and she didn't call 911, she just abandoned me, and now I am in a wheelchair, crippled for life. As a kid, no one ever helped me with my homework, no one said, when you get your period, here's what you do. I don't even know what a family is. I have cried and cried and been very, very sad. But now I am really trying to find happiness and hang onto it, and not be that way. But it's hard." Tears had come into Vivian's eyes as she spoke.

I repeated back to Vivian everything she had said, asking "Do I have this right?" as she nodded. I wanted to honor her feelings of abandonment, desperation, sadness, and debility, as well as her initiative to find happiness. I felt heartsick that Vivian felt "crippled for life." It was a power-ful narrative, but from my work with Maeli and Alexis and Elena, I didn't think it was true.

"Your efforts to try to find happiness, I am wondering if you've seen any tiny signs of being able to do that?"

"Yeah," Vivian said. "I've seen some improvements." Some days she felt okay, and suicide wasn't on her mind anymore.

"You know, one thing I have learned in my work is the capacity of the human spirit for healing. Those improvements you've noticed, I am won-dering if maybe they would be a sign that you are *not* crippled for life."

"I hope so. That's what I want for myself."

A few weeks later, Vivian's therapist told her she was leaving for a new job. Vivian didn't show for her next appointment with me, and didn't respond to my phone calls. I understood her reluctance. We had not proven to be reliably present for her. Every few weeks, I called her and left a message, and finally, three months later, she came to see me, in September of her senior year.

"I'm still not over the abortion," she said. As usual, she was dressed in an understated, effortlessly fashionable outfit. We had established that I would be able to see her weekly for psychotherapy, and Vivian was grateful. "It was a living person," Vivian went on. "I'm sad about it." She looked at me discerningly. "I talk to her. Do you think that is weird?"

"Not at all," I said. "What do you talk to her about?"

"Everything. She is a source of inspiration for me."

"In what way does she inspire you?"

"She's like a reference for me, reminding me how I want to be. Joy, that's what I've named her." Vivian paused. "I have been thinking about the rape."

"Uh huh," I said. "What about it?"

"I have three ex-boyfriends. And I noticed that in that past, if I didn't want to have sex with them, I still did. And that has me thinking, the day of the incident with my cousin, I did not want it to happen—he proba-bly—I don't remember exactly what happened. I wish I knew. But what I noticed was that I do that a lot, I really want to say no but I am not able to say it. Anthony, the kid who got me pregnant—the things I allowed him to do to me. I want to be able to say no. I want complete control of myself and to say what I want to say."

"You want to say what you want to say."

"Yes. I want to own who I am." Vivian looked quietly resolute. "I've started applying to law school. I've finished six applications already. It's my vision for my life, to be an advocate for people. I want to work hard, help people, get an apartment, decorate it the way I want, live my life the way I want."

"You want to live your life the way you want."

"Yes. I am trying to not get so upset about things or text boys that I don't want to text or have sex when I don't want to have sex. I want to complete the circle of me being me."

During these appointments, I focused on forging a connection with Vivian and helping her develop her sources of inspiration, her values, her intentions, her preferred ways of soothing herself, and a community that truly supported her. In narrative practice, helping someone deal with traumatic experiences begins with bringing forward narratives of who the person is and what they value, and with practices that promote well-being and connection with people who are loving and trustworthy. Not only are these elements a prerequisite for speaking about trauma in ways that are therapeutic, they are the essence—the *point*—of healing from trauma.

Trauma is traumatic because it desecrates what people hold precious and blocks their sense of agency to act in accordance with their values. This breach disrupts the processes of consciousness and memory that allow each of us to know who we are with a sense of continuity and integrity. Trauma corrodes a coherent narrative of self. It leads people to feel "I am not myself" and to lose touch with who that preferred self might be.

More severe trauma has even more severe effects. John Stillman, in his *Narrative Therapy Trauma Manual,*[2] distills the work of Lev Vygotsky, Russell Meares, and Michael White in describing what happens: More severe trauma leads to further disruption of consciousness and memory, leading to loss of awareness of who one has been over time, or autobiographical memory, with difficulty incorporating new experiences into the story of one's life. Even more severe trauma disrupts the working memory that enables us to know what to do in response to new life events, and at its worst, trauma leads to the loss of a sense of what is real and what is not. With each of these effects, the memory of the trauma and its effects increasingly dominate the person's experience.

Therefore, one of the primary tasks in helping someone recover from trauma is to support the restoration of a sense of self—the feeling "I am myself" that arises when people understand what they value and hold the intention to act in accordance with those values. Restoration of this narrative of personal identity is the basis for further recovery from trauma. As Stillman puts it, as "intentionality gets reestablished, individuals reconnect with the ability to make decisions in their lives, so they can examine the effects of trauma and events can be characterized in ways not supported by trauma and in support of what is valued. The effects of trauma are then reduced."[3]

In working with trauma, we are engaged in what Michael White calls "doubly listening." He writes:

> In my work with people who have been through trauma, it's very important that I not only hear whatever it is that is important for them to share about the story of trauma, but that I also provide a foundation through my questions that gives people an opportunity to resurrect and to further develop a preferred "sense of self" and to identify how they responded to the trauma they were being put through…. No one is the passive recipient of trauma. People always take steps to try to prevent the trauma, and, even if preventing the trauma is clearly impossible, they take steps to try to modify its effects on their lives, or they take steps to preserve what is precious to them.[4]

In my work with Vivian, I was listening to hear whatever she wanted to tell me of her experiences of trauma *and* I was listening for how she had resisted trauma and held onto what was precious to her despite trauma.

## Honoring Both Grief/Pain/Fear/Loss and Strength/Agency/Meaning/Identity When Treating Trauma

Witnessing with compassion what, if anything, the person wishes to share about the trauma they experienced, including grief, pain, fear, or loss

AND

Listening for and developing stories of strength, agency, meaning, and identity in the face of trauma:

Intentions to survive, recover, and/or thrive despite the trauma

Acts of resistance or protest, however small or internal

What experiences of pain or loss are a testimony to

Successes in holding onto cherished values

Skills of self-soothing

Connections with others

Drawing on healing communities and cultural traditions

Activism

The meaning of these actions for the person's identity

What each person needs to heal from trauma is different, and different at different times. Individuals and cultures have developed many effective ways to deal with disastrous or horrific life events.[5] In working with people who have experienced trauma, it behooves us to honor their personal preferences and cultural traditions of responding to and recovering from devastating life events, rather than imposing a particular "debriefing" or treatment approach. When we listen closely to what people say about how they tried to prevent trauma, how they survived, and what they find healing, we can prioritize their own values and skills. In eliciting people's stories of survival and recovery, we can strengthen their connections to the people and traditions that they find most supportive and meaningful.

Trauma often occurs in contexts in which powerful discourses of privilege and oppression are operating, such as racism or sexism. Judiciously naming and exposing the influences of these discourses can decrease trauma survivors' experiences of isolation and negative self-worth and offer possibilities for connection with a valued community and positive identity development.

In addition to our patients' personal and cultural resources, we can collaboratively consider with our patients whether any of the trauma treatments in our psychiatric tool kit might be helpful to them, such as Somatic Experiencing® and eye-movement desensitization and reprocessing. The key addition that narrative practices offers to trauma treatment is the continuous development of the story of resistance and holding onto precious values and relationships in the face of trauma. This lost story of strength and meaning not only powerfully supports recovery; at times it is so healing that it makes other types of trauma treatments unnecessary.[6]

Vivian missed her next appointment with me, but came in two weeks later, and weekly after that. Vivian herself titrated how much we spoke about the rape and its impact on her life. I "doubly listened" for both what was painful and for how she had kept her spirit alive. The conversations that follow took place over several meetings that fall.

"There is so much power we have in ourselves that we are not aware of," she said, speaking about a trip she took by herself.

"How did you come to that conclusion?" I asked.

"Before Joy, I wanted to be independent, but I wasn't. After I had Joy I realized that I need to be good at this. I can't have her looking at me like I am a loser. I want her to be proud of me. Like when my mom was creating problems with me and my sister, I didn't let that affect me."

"So you noticed this ability you have…?"

"Of not letting things get to me."

"And how do you do that?"

"Okay. Like on my econ exam, I didn't do well, I wanted to leave and cry, but I pictured Joy talking to me, saying, 'It's okay.' With my sister and mom, that's what I did. Joy said, 'It's okay. That is how they are. They are not going to change.'"

"You have this ability to keep Joy alive in your life."

Vivian looked self-conscious, and I saw that I had missed the mark, both spiritually and culturally. "I know she is dead," she said quietly, "but her spirit is alive. I believe that when we die, our spirit is somewhere, alive."

"Her spirit is alive and inspires you," I said, following what she said more closely, seeking to repair my misstep. The last thing I wanted to do was to diminish this precious source of inspiration in her life.

"Yes. I have Joy and I have God, and I have been living in a way that Joy and God would be happy with me."

"And what kind of way is that?"

"Like a mom, as if I were someone's mom. I have to discipline myself. No one wants her mother to be sloppy." We nodded together in understanding. Vivian took on a look of determination. "I want to have Joy see me like I see my grandmother." Vivian described her grandmother as the one person who offered her unconditional love. In creating her connection with Joy, Vivian was keeping the mutual love and admiration she shared with her grandmother more present in her life.

At a subsequent meeting she said, "I am on this new journey. I take time for myself. I don't let anything distract me from what is most important to me: first, finishing my education, and then doing work that makes a difference."

"You are on a new journey, going toward what is most important to you."

"Yes. I'm not going to have sex if I don't want to. I like how I am creating my life. When I think of the rape, I used to lie in bed in the dark all day and cry, but now when I think of it, I lie in bed for an hour watching TV, and then I get up and get on with my life."

In December, Vivian came in saying she was feeling a bit down. "I got rejected from a law school in New York, and I thought, *If I don't get in, life is over*, and then I thought, *If I don't get in, I don't want things to go downhill*, and I realized, I am doing better, I am trusting God, I have Joy, whatever direction life takes me, I will find a way, I always find a way."

"You will find a way. Can you tell me about another time when you found a way, when things were hard?" I asked.

"After I got the abortion, I was still stuck in the same dorm complex as that kid, and then in the psych ward I was a mess, but I found a way. I moved to a new dorm across campus in a suite with my friends and I eliminated the boy from my life. Even as a kid, I found a way."

"How did you find a way, when you were a kid?"

Vivian sighed. "In Ghana, they moved me around a lot, after that time when my uncle called me a witch and kicked me out of his home." Vivian spoke of how painful it was that no one supported her as they moved her around from house to house, not even her parents, concluding with, "And I got out of that situation, too."

"How did you do it?"

"I went to live with my sister, even though I had to totally take care of myself. No one ever even said to me, 'This is how you brush your teeth.'"

"But you did it."

"I survived. That's my password: survivor1991." Vivian sighed. "It's easier now, because I have God and Joy. I know what I am worth now."

You can hear in this conversation how I am cultivating the story "I always find a way" in the context of her traumatic experiences. This story of her strength and determination in the face of trauma promotes an awareness of personal agency and a positive sense of self that the trauma might have robbed her of. In doing this piece of work, we are acknowledging and grieving what was painful about the trauma, and we are simultaneously honoring Vivian's determination and ingenuity to find her way forward to a better life.

I didn't see Vivian for the month over winter break, and when she returned, she said, "I am doing well this year. Things have changed. I am more disciplined, I do my work on time, go to sleep by ten, I am more goal-oriented. Nothing is going to stop me from making a life in which I can be somebody." She was attending all her classes. There was someone she had briefly dated at age sixteen who was still interested in her.

"Mark is good to me and I enjoy his company," she said, "But it's better for me not to have sex." She had been able to tell him that and stick to it. "I noticed that I have the power to voice what I want and what I need."

"Wow," I said, taking notes as usual, and repeating Vivian's words back to her as I did so. "You have the power—to voice—what you want—and what you need."

"I have my own voice."

"You have your own voice. And how is that for you?"

"It's great." Vivian smiled.

At our next appointments, Vivian continued with this theme. She said, "When I was raped, I was feeling then so scared and alone. I didn't have my own voice. But now I have learned to have my own voice and I am able to speak up." We spoke of her past and present successes in speaking up. "Whenever I feel the moment that I want to speak up, I feel strong. In my heart, I am connected to Joy. A beautiful strength woke up here," she said, touching her heart.

"Joy woke up something in you," I said.

"Definitely. When I was in high school, I wanted to be strong, but I wasn't there yet. I fell down whenever I was with a guy. I wanted to be somebody, to be independent and happy, but I wasn't there yet."

"Now you are."

"Yes. I feel more at peace nowadays. I'm not fighting with anything inside of me."

In our work together that spring, Vivian and I celebrated how far she had come and the daily well-being that she was experiencing. Suicidal urges were entirely absent, and Vivian was proud of her grades in her classes and how she was managing her relationships. I was grateful and delighted, but I was also aware that she was preparing to graduate in May, say good-bye to me, and go out into the world on her own. I wanted her to be well-prepared and well-provisioned. Over the course of our last two months of work together, we continued to develop the story of her strengths, successes, hopes, and dreams. I wrote down the things she said and created a letter that I gave to her. We spoke about my writing this book, and she said she was happy to have the story of our work together be part of it.

At one of our last meetings, I asked her what she would take with her from our work together. She said, "What I will take from this room is that I can't go back to my old ways; it's not an option. My purpose is to keep growing. The way I talk and act is different now. I know I will never have anyone treat me like that, how I used to let boys treat me. I am worth more than that." She said that Joy continued to be a source of inspiration. "I talk to her and act in a way that pleases her." Vivian looked thoughtful. "It's like I am mothering myself, and I know how to do that. I know that if I want to change, if I don't put the effort in, it won't happen." Through Joy, Vivian kept alive the love, both gentle and firm, that she learned from her grandmother, a love that she could offer to herself, mothering herself.

At our last visit, I asked Vivian to tell me the highlights of her time at college. Here is what she said:

> I found who I am.
> I speak up in relationships.
> I am stronger emotionally.
> I pamper myself.
> I do what makes me happy.
> If I am sad, I get up and keep moving.
> If something bad happens, I hold onto the bigger picture of
>     what I am trying to fulfill so I can keep going.
> If I have inner peace, everything else will go well.
> God is important.
> When I am a mother, I want to have a close relationship with
>     my kids.
> I will never give up on myself.
> I have to fulfill the purpose I have in life.
> I have met people who have been helpful.
> It feels so good to have the power to speak up about what
>     I want and what I don't want.

## VIVIAN'S REFLECTIONS

Six months after our last visit, Vivian sent me an e-mail to catch me up on how she was:

> I am doing good so far. I am still trying to work on my relationship with God. These days it's all about God, Joy and me. My relationship with my mom is getting a little better. She offered to help me with rent but I told her, no it's okay. I realized that if I were my mother I would not want to have this kind of relationship with Joy or want Joy to keep holding things in so I try to be nice to her and not let her get to me. Joy has taught me so much and given me this inner strength I never thought I had.
>
> I am still in a relationship with Martin and still practicing abstinence. I am in a relationship with him but my world does not evolve around him nor neither would I say am in love with him. I like him but I am taking things very slow with him emotional-wise. Relationships are tough because when I was single it was so much easier to just live how I want and not be bother with anyone or become weak or vulnerable. In a relationship, you do like the person and you do care about them so you have to be careful you do not fall too deep and lose your sense of self. I am not perfect either, every now and then he might do something that will make me super sad when I really need not to be sad. When that happens I assess the situation and if it's something that I overacted I apologize and if its something he did that I did not like I will tell him. We try to practice good communication and so far things have been good between us. We go on dates once in a while, he helps me out if I really need help and he does not pressure me with sex but we both are taking things slow.
>
> If I did not have Joy I probably would not be as strong as I am today. I am still applying for schools, I am not allowing some boy to come sweep me off and lose my sense of self, I am able to speak out and tell him what I do not like or like. I am still working on myself but so far I am happy with where I am.

## Notes

1. Thanks to Jenifer McKenna, Gerry Weiss, Jeffrey Fishman, and Beth Prullage for teaching me this form.
2. John Stillman, *Narrative Therapy Trauma Manual: A Principle-Based Approach* (St. Louis Park, MN: Casperson, 2012), 57–69.
3. Stillman, *Trauma Manual,* 69.
4. Michael White, "Working with People Who Are Suffering the Consequences of Multiple Trauma: A Narrative Perspective," *The International Journal of Narrative Therapy and Community Work* 1 (2004), 48.
5. See, for example, Ethan Watters, *Crazy Like Us: The Globalization of the American Psyche* (New York: Free Press, 2010), 65–126.
6. Ncube, "The Tree of Life," 3–16.

# CHAPTER NINE

# Finding Happiness

*Rising from Despair and Turning
Away from Anxiety*

"Anxiety is ruining my life," Addie Markiewicz had said to me at her first appointment at age sixteen. Now, four years later, she entered my office, dropped her backpack on the floor, plopped down comfortably on the couch, picked up one of my blue throw pillows and began fiddling with the zipper. A junior in college, Addie had long, dark hair, blue eyes, fair skin, wholesome good looks, and a dry, at times mischievous sense of humor. In our weekly sessions, she could be alternately reticent and forthcoming. A gifted student with lots of friends, she volunteered at a daycare facility for children with special needs and was a respected and beloved babysitter for several families in the area. She had helped to form an advocacy group at her college for students who were dealing with mental health challenges. She had a loving relationship with her parents, whom she called her "best friends," and her life had been free of any major trauma; on the contrary, her childhood had been characterized by a loving, supportive family and a close-knit community of which she was a cherished member, many of whom shared her Polish American heritage.

For the first three years of our work together, I met with Addie for twenty minutes every week or two and she also met with a psychotherapist. After he moved out of the area, I became her primary psychotherapist, meeting with her weekly for fifty minutes. She had made great strides in overcoming profound despair, an ongoing sense of unreality, severe anxiety, and unwanted compulsive urges that had dogged her since she was twelve, but at times one or more of these problems flared up again, and we were still chipping away at them, working toward a fuller recovery. From our first appointment, she had identified a problem of feeling an overwhelming urge to spend hours and hours on her homework until it was flawless, accompanied by a keen anxiety lest there were any mistakes. In the course of our conversations, she named this problem "perfectionism," and while she had successfully reduced its impact on her life, it was still more influential than she wished.

In this chapter, I will describe my work with Addie in the fourth year of her treatment with me, focusing on our efforts to achieve the fullest possible remission of her symptoms to make way for well-being, and if possible, joy.

## UNPACKING PERFECTIONISM

Addie began her weekly session by speaking about some of her successes in not following the dictates of perfectionism. "I am starting to have time for things other than homework. I just wrote my homework without rereading it or adding any extra ideas and today I turned it in. Then I wrote my paper for my children's literature class on two books. I wrote it all out in one sitting and it didn't flow that well but I finished it and decided I was not going to stress out about the bibliography." She said that then she was able to spend time with her friends.

I asked her what steps she was taking to make this more possible, and she said she had developed a strategy where she limited the time she did homework. "I give myself blocks of time where I can do one thing and block out other stuff, like worries about procrastination. When I do homework, I just do homework, and when I am with my friends, I am just with my friends."

"What might be a name for this strategy?" I asked. My intention was to highlight this skill and make it more available to use again.

"Blocking," she said. "Previously, I had filled all my free time with homework."

"But now you are using blocking, so you can do what you want with your free time."

"Yes. It's like I am de-anchoring the boat. So the boat can be free to sail around. I am the sailor, and I had been anchored and secure with perfectionism, but now using blocking...."

"You can sail about more as you prefer."

"Yes."

"And how is that for you?" I asked.

"I like it better when everyone in the room knows that I'm the best. Because I am always going to be the best. I am always going to know the most. Then I'm in control and I know what to expect."

"What do you mean?" I asked.

"Then I am immune to consequences and getting yelled at. For example, sometimes in class teachers yell. The teacher is yelling at the whole class, but it feels like she is just yelling at me, unless I do the work perfectly." Addie put down the pillow she was holding and picked up a little basket of stones and shells that I keep on a shelf. She sorted through the basket's contents and chose a sand dollar to hold in her hand, setting the basket back on the shelf. She had actually given me that sand dollar several years earlier.

It's common for a problem like perfectionism to induce anxiety when someone succeeds in resisting it, or even talks about resisting it, which was what was happening in our session. It was an opportunity to unpack the perfectionism further to reveal how it was operating and give Addie more traction in her efforts. As mentioned in chapter 5, to expose the wily ways of problems, we can use the therapeutic strategy of thinking about the problem as a person who can be interrogated.

"So how would you characterize your relationship with perfectionism, if perfectionism was a person?" I asked.

"I want to be his best friend," she said. "Then I will be safe."

"Safe in what way?"

"Safe from even a little crack of not being in control."

"Would you say perfectionism is making a claim that you have to always be in control?"

"Yes. If you are in control, you must be sane. Perfectionism lets me be in control and that's how I know I have my sanity." Addie tapped the sand dollar against her chin.

Knowing she had her sanity was particularly salient to Addie. When she first met with me at age sixteen, she was afraid she was losing her mind. Her previous psychiatrist had been unhelpful, and after two months with me, she dropped out of treatment entirely, returning to see me six months later with symptoms of anxiety, depression, and unreality that were dramatically worse. For the first three years of our work together, when she was in high school and the first year of college, despite her dedication to meet with me and try treatments, Addie's symptoms improved only incrementally. School, work, and sports became impossible. Suicidal thoughts were constant. I worried we might lose her to suicide, and inquired about suicide at every appointment, but no matter how strong the suicidal thoughts were, what was stronger was her desire not to cause pain to her parents by taking her life. When she became fatigued in resisting suicidal urges, she let me know and we used voluntary psychiatric hospitalization to provide support.

Here is how Addie describes those years:

Life before finding the right support and experiencing healing was horrid. I did not express how terrified I constantly felt, so because there was such a discrepancy between how I appeared and how I felt, it was hard to be taken as seriously as I needed to be. While I did initially try to explain my feelings of unreality with others, I gave up early on due to not feeling like words could capture the terror. As the years went on, I felt like more and more strings that connected me to reality were breaking and I spent the majority of my time obsessing about losing my mind. My mind sometimes gave me a break from insanity concerns and instead focused on creating and maintaining obsessions revolving around death. There were many experiences I had in middle school and high school where at the end of the day I thought to myself, "Wow that would have been really fun if only I wasn't depressed."

Every day was a constant battle between deciding if I wanted to leave my room and face unbearable anxiety or if I wanted to stay home and feel depressed. I experienced depression as an incredibly unbearable sense of anguish that always circled around my body until the core was totally affected, at which point I felt so incapacitated that I did not have a will to live. The isolation of knowing that no one had even the tiniest inkling of what was going on in my mind, made everything worse. I justified suicide by stating that death will eventually happen for all of us. I also became obsessed with the idea that the only thing that could save me from this hell was being perfect. This plan did not work for me unfortunately. I was concerned by the way people would look at me when I talked to them, so I often wrote down my miseries. One of the most illustrative journal entries of how I felt during this time was written at age 17. "Good people are happy and bad people are depressed. Some people have lives that are wonderful. Some people have lives that are decent. And some people have lives where all they want to do is kill themselves over and over again day after day after day. And that is the kind of life I have. It's just not worth it. Nothing is worth it."

Throughout this time of life-threatening symptoms, I worked with Addie to both honor her anguish and to seek to gradually dismantle her symptoms. We used every resource we could think of to help her, including partial hospitalization programs and trials of a wide range of medications, including antipsychotics and mood stabilizers, ultimately finding two that she felt were consistently beneficial, citalopram and lamotrigine. Addie was a tireless advocate for herself, and she found and consulted with a specialist in de-realization[1] who recommended the lamotrigine, which helped reduce the sense of unreality but did not eliminate it. She had an uncle who had schizophrenia, and given the intensity of her feelings of unreality and the way that symptoms were disrupting her life, we were concerned that she was also developing schizophrenia. Experts in that field thought it likely when we consulted with them,[2] but as years passed, she has not developed any significant psychotic symptoms. She saw also saw a specialist who ruled out temporal lobe epilepsy. Very gradually over the four years we worked together, using all that narrative psychiatry had to offer, Addie's symptoms improved to the point that they were no longer dominating her life.

So to return to our conversation four years into treatment, it was no wonder that the narrative that perfectionism was necessary for her to feel sane was a powerful one, and particularly important to unpack.

I asked Addie, "So perfectionism is saying that it is a way for you to know that you have your sanity?"

"The only way." Addie put the sand dollar back and picked up a pillow again, fuchsia this time.

"That's what perfectionism is saying," I said, "but I am wondering if there are other times that you feel a sense of your sanity, when perfectionism isn't present?"

Addie took a deep breath. "Yes, going to Cape Cod with Janice last weekend. I was able to just have a good time."

"Tell me more about that." We spoke about what they did at the beach and how that made her feel, and then I said, "So perfectionism is making this claim that it's necessary for your sanity, but it appears that that's not true. What do you think?"

"I agree. But it feels like it's true." Addie turned the pillow end over end in her hands.

"It's not true, but it feels true. Our time is almost up for today, but we can talk more about this next time."

"Can you write down the big philosophical ideas that we discussed so I can remember them?"

"Of course." I wrote out direct quotes of what Addie had said, about the usefulness of blocking, sailing where she wanted, feeling sanity when she was with Janice, and that the claims of perfectionism were not true, retelling and strengthening the new narratives she was creating.

## TREASURED VALUES AS A POTENT FORCE

The following week, after Addie settled in, we again took up the question of perfectionism and sanity.

"I feel a connection to sanity when I am with Janice. And also when everything around me is clean and organized, then I feel I have my sanity," she said. "My mind untwists. Organizing is comforting. I like having the right folders for the right classes, I like making lists. But then perfectionism can happen easier." Addie picked up the fuchsia pillow from the corner of the couch.

"Organizing is comforting, but it makes perfectionism happen more easily?"

"Perfectionism—it's really more for others. Organizing, that's more for me."

"Organizing is more for you?"

Here we were refining the boundaries of the problem.

"Organizing's not a problem," said Addie. "It's the perfectionism that's the problem. It tells me I have to be perfect at school and with other people."

"Perfectionism is making claims about school and other people?"

"Yes, that I need to do things perfectly to keep my sanity."

"What does it say that you are able to experience a sense of sanity in other ways, like with Janice?" Here I invited Addie to articulate the *meaning* of the examples she had given about ways she experienced sanity without perfectionism.

"Being perfect is not necessary," Addie said.

"Being perfect is not necessary," I repeated, in a tiny retelling of this new narrative.

Addie opened and closed the zipper on the pillow. "I can't handle being perfect all the time. It feels like it's not a choice, but I am so tired from trying to be perfect. I am burnt out."

"You are burnt out from trying to be perfect," I said. Addie nodded. "And you have had some success in resisting perfectionism, like not spending as much time on your homework."

"I want to do more variety of things not perfectly," she said.

"Like what?"

"Like not answer every question the teacher asks."

"And have you tried that?"

"Yes. It was nerve-wracking. Because I knew the answers. And everyone knew that I knew."

"So how did you coach yourself to be able to do that?"

"I paid less attention in class, and I thought of what happens when I'm not at class."

"And in paying less attention in class, and in thinking of what happens when you're not there, you were able to resist perfectionism?"

"A bit. Even if I can't completely give up control, I can give up a little control. Everything in life is not all or nothing."

Addie had made a statement that could serve as an overarching theme or even a moral for the new narrative we were creating. I strengthened the power of her statement by repeating it and by offering it a title.

"Everything in life is not all or nothing. Would you say that that is an anti-perfectionism saying?"

"Yes. It's good to go against perfectionism."

"Why is it good?"

Asking *Why?* invited Addie to reflect on her values, permitting us to compare them with the effects of the problem, a juxtaposition that can be galvanizing.

"Because," Addie said, setting the pillow in her lap and looking toward the corner of the room, "perfectionism is this one thing in life that affects a lot of things—in ways that are not obvious. Because of spending all this time on homework, I just don't spend a lot of time listening and empathizing with others. When I think about that it makes me feel worse. I am not involved with others' lives and stories. It's unbalanced—people tell me things and I can't remember what they say. I had always thought that my problems were worse than other people's, but now I know they are not always worse."

"It has felt unbalanced. You have wanted to be able to listen to and empathize with others more."

"Yes."

"It's something you really care about, something that perfectionism got in the way of. What is it like to realize this?"

"I feel bad. I wasted years inside my mind. I have been trying to make it more balanced for a long time."

"When did you first start to try to make it more balanced?"

"The year that Deedee's brother died, back when we were seniors in high school. She was so down and never wanted to see any of us. I had known her since kindergarten and I was trying to figure out how to reach out to her. But I couldn't do it." The beginnings of tears came into Addie's eyes. "I want to be able to put aside my feelings to help someone else."

"You want to be able to help someone else." Tears came into my eyes as well.

"That was three years ago. She's okay now, but I feel guilty about it."

"Three years ago the perfectionism was really dominating your life. Depression, too," I said. "You were putting all your energy into just staying alive."

Addie nodded.

"But what you really care about is being able to help someone else. You would like to be able to be more true to that, and not let perfectionism get in the way of that."

Addie nodded again.

"And has there been a time when you have been able to help someone a bit, despite perfectionism?"

"That weekend on Cape Cod, with Janice, I was able to get out of my own mind and be there for her. I was able to stop her and stop me from worrying at the same time. We both had homework due, but we were able to not study when we were on Cape Cod."

Addie compellingly articulated a value that was precious to her, of wanting to be able to help others, and how she did not want perfectionism to stop her from doing that. Our patients' deepest values are one of the most potent forces that can be harnessed to help them overcome their problems.

We can anticipate that whenever we generate a new narrative that contradicts the narrative associated with the problem, the old narrative will reassert itself. Questioning the personified problem is a particularly incisive way to reveal problem-promoting rhetoric and prepare our patients to resist it. So I asked, "How does perfectionism respond when you take these kind of steps?"

"It gets madder. But now when I am resisting it more, there are only limited times that it is stronger. So I can get rid of it."

"Is there any role in your life for perfectionism?"

"When I am writing prescriptions," she said, and looked at me with a wry smile. Months ago when we were speaking about perfectionism, we had discussed the role of perfectionism and the limited times it might be helpful, and I had mentioned writing prescriptions as a rare time that perfectionism was helpful to me, since prescriptions need to be exactly correct. Addie went on, "But not in my life. My goal is to not be thinking one hundred percent of the time. I am usually thinking about thinking, and I want things to just happen."

"Would you like me to write anything about what we spoke about today?"

"No. What I want are questions, questions like what you ask."

"Ok," I said, took out a clean sheet of paper, and wrote the following questions, to invite the development of lost stories of strength:

- In what ways are you resisting perfectionism today?

- What moments of freedom from perfectionism have you had?

- Your value of being there for others, how might someone see that in your life this week?

- What did you have to overcome to keep this commitment to be there for others?

At the beginning of our next meeting, Addie was somber and reticent. She said the anxiety, depression, and unreality were worse. The good things about perfectionism were on her mind. She noted that she first developed perfectionism at age twelve, after she had had a serious depression, and she said that depression and perfectionism were "on different teams, but worked together."

Then Addie said, "The problem is that I have learned how to not be depressed. So the depression is confused, it doesn't understand that it's over. When the depression was there, I was numb. Now I cry and cry and cry about things to be sad about. I can be sad about sad things. Now it's good that I can feel something."

It appeared to me that Addie was recovering from depression and perfectionism, and she was grieving the impact they had had on her life. My sense was that she was in a liminal space, a space of transition in which she had moved away from depression and perfectionism, but had not yet fully cultivated the things in her life that the absence of depression and perfectionism made room for.[3]

At the end of this meeting, Addie again asked for questions to take with her. I focused this time on eliciting stories of both love and happiness.

- If there was a team that was in favor of Addie's happiness, what kinds of experiences would it be in favor of?

- Who are the boosters for this team?

- What that is important to Addie would this team be promoting?

At our next meeting, Addie said she was feeling "a little anxious, but not much" and was not depressed, but was feeling happy, due to a combination of factors: not thinking over and over what she has to do, doing less homework on the weekend, and increasing her exercise. She said, "I am so close to being better." She had written out answers to the questions, which she read to me and we expanded upon, a sampling of which follows:

If there was a team that was in favor of Addie's happiness, what kinds of experiences would it be in favor of?
*Going back to gymnastics* ("I want to take all Saturday off as a 'fun day' and do stuff like jump on the trampoline, which brings

me joy"), *doing stuff during the weekday besides school related stuff* ("like getting my nose pierced with friends, I'll put that on the top of my list and homework lower on my list"), *doing things more spontaneously* ("on weekends I want to be more at ease when there is a change of plans"), *seeing/talking to high school friends more* ("like Deedee, who I saw on Sunday"), *dream bulletin board* ("everything I want symbolized"), *not punishing myself after missed classes* ("still doing fun stuff on weekdays anyways"), *and taking Spunky for ice cream* (her dog, "before he dies.")

Who are the boosters for this team?

*Connie and Tim* (her parents), *Deedee and Janice* (friends), *Bruce and Paul* (friends from college; "they make you not think and just have fun"), *Raphael and Lionel* ("my advisor and professor from the psych department, they are nice and calm and know how to have fun and they make me do fun stuff'), *Full Circle peoples* (the kids at the day care where she volunteered); *and also the kids I babysit for.*

What that is important to Addie would this team be promoting? *A stressless life.*

Throughout these four sessions, you can hear how we investigated the perfectionism as if it were a person influencing Addie's life. This is a therapeutic strategy that helps to weaken a problem by exposing, questioning, and, at times, discounting the narratives that strengthen the problem, narratives like, "I need to do things perfectly to maintain my sanity." When the intentions and values of the problem's narratives are made overt, then the patient is able to contrast them with her own intentions and values, such as Addie becoming clear that her value of helping other people was more important to her than perfectionism's value of doing homework perfectly. At first clarifying this led Addie to experience heightened anxiety and sadness as she grieved the ways that perfectionism had drawn her away from some of her most precious intentions, but ultimately it paved the way for her to more fully commit to creating "a stressless life" that included fun, friendship, and joy.

## GENERATING NARRATIVES OF HAPPINESS

Over the ensuing months, we continued to develop the narrative of what Addie valued and what she wanted in her life in the space made available by the absence of depression and perfectionism. I offered her questions at the end of our sessions, for which she wrote answers that she shared with me at our next meeting. She noted that she preferred questions addressed in the third person. Here are some of the questions I gave her over several sessions, for which she gave me detailed answers:

In what ways is Addie using creativity to bring herself support nowadays?

Are there kinds of support that Addie would like to bring forward more?

When does Addie feel most at ease?

What makes Addie laugh?

What would be nice for Addie to do for fun on school days?

What would be fun for Addie to do over Thanksgiving?

As we addressed these questions, Addie began asking a question of identity: *Who am I without depression and anxiety?* She said that she felt that there was a discontinuity in her identity. "There's who I was before the depression and then there was the depression when I lost everything. And that is so painful I don't even want to think about it." She leaned over to dig around in her backpack and brought out a small clump of plastic grapes, which she turned over in her hands.

"If we could find some continuity, would that be helpful to you?" I asked.

"Sure. But there isn't anything."

"I'm thinking about how much you care about children. Might that be an example of something you valued when you were young and also now?""

Yes. I just got my schedule at Full Circle for next semester."

"What is it that you value about working there?"

"I love children."

"Why is that?"

"They are so cute and little."

"When might someone have first noticed your love of children?"

"When I was twelve, I babysat a six-month-old, and I fed him," Addie said, warming to her subject and speaking with animation, "and it was the greatest experience, because he was so cute, and it was right across the street, and I got money for it."

"What was his name?"

"Brandon."

We went on to speak of other babysitting experiences, and how she parlayed that into her volunteer work with disabled children at Full Circle and the hopes she had to become a teacher, possibly in special education. In addition to the suffering she had experienced, Addie felt that she had lost much from the severity of the depression and anxiety: a chance to go to an elite college, play college varsity sports, have fun in high school, and to simply do the ordinary developmental tasks of late adolescence. Finding ways in which she had kept precious aspects of herself alive through that time honored her tenacity and integrity and helped her create an adult identity that felt grounded in her life.

A few months later, Addie, who was increasingly full of creative ideas for supporting her well-being, brought in her "note card project." She settled herself on my couch and pulled a pack of 3-by-5 cards out of her backpack. "Everyday I write 'why the day was successful' on the front and 'conclusions' on the back." She smiled. "This is very you-ish."

"Very me-ish? What do you mean?"

"Just listen." Addie took the top card from the pack and read it. "Yesterday was successful because I went to Zumba *and* I modified the parts that were too hard. And my conclusion was," she turned over the card, "I can modify something instead of giving up, which is pro-effort and con-perfectionism."

"Wow!" I said. "I wonder if that applies to other situations as well?"

"Yes," said Addie. "I am using it to tweak my response to perfectionism. Want to hear another?"

"Absolutely."

Addie took a fresh card from her deck. "February 4. Today was successful because I babysat a three-month-old, which was the first time I had babysat someone so young, and he slept the whole time. Conclusion: It's another thing to add to the list that fears are worse than the actual experience."

She went on to read:

"Feb. 6. Today was successful because my abstract on test anxiety was picked to be presented at a psychology conference. Conclusion: This is good, because I want to study anxiety.

"Feb. 5. Today was successful because even though I was beyond depleted and in bed at 4 pm, I still went out with friends and it was perfectly tolerable. Conclusion: Depression tried to rope me down, but I prevailed because I stopped thinking about the abstract and focused on doing something concrete.

"Feb 2. Amanda and I got second place in a cake contest. Conclusion: Doing stuff is fun. You can compete in a lighthearted way. Fun is as important as academics.

"Feb 1. Today was successful because I stayed through an entire 75-minute class. Conclusion: One symptom during one time period does not guarantee that the symptom will last all day.

"Jan 31. Today was successful because I developed a new homework strategy of putting a time limit on how long I spent on one assignment. Conclusion: Being innovative helps with the anti-perfectionism crusade."

Addie smiled at me comfortably. All on her own, she was creating healing and empowering narratives that supported her well-being. These narratives included the landscape of action—successful events—and the landscape of meaning—her conclusions, the meanings Addie gave those events. Addie was not only creating narratives that supported her well-being; she was creating *methods for generating* such narratives.

I sighed and smiled. I felt great gratitude. Addie had reclaimed her life, and anxiety and depression were no longer ruining it. She had found happiness.

## ADDIE'S REFLECTIONS

The first time I had a panic attack, I thought I entered heaven. I was walking between my parents through a parking lot after

I had left my 6th grade basketball game and the snow around me was circling around in a huge white veil. I have a distinct memory of the moment I thought my feet left the ground and I began to float through the spinning white world in complete amazement that something could be so white.

Four months after that first panic attack, I met a psychiatrist for the first time. He spoke to my parents for the majority of the consultation, and I began to wonder if he had forgotten I was present in the room. The next four years with this psychiatrist were extremely tiresome as every few months my parents and I would visit him for fifteen minutes and leave with more questions than answers. This doctor typically laughed at my answers to his questions, refused to meet with me privately, even for a couple minutes for the entire four years, and never attempted to explain any portion of my treatment with me.

My first impression of Dr. Hamkins was that she was too human to be a psychiatrist. I became very nervous during the time we regularly met in the beginning that there was actually hope for me, because I wanted to keep my identity as a person who had an illness defined by terror. I wanted this not because I was enjoying this life, but because I spent great amounts of effort learning to adjust and cope with this way of life that I feared the work I knew would be involved to get better. In response to an inquiry from a friend of why I would not return to Dr. Hamkins after my break from all psychological treatment, I wrote in an email, "There was absolutely nothing I liked about her, except that she was really compassionate, and actually listened to me, and made me feel safe. I'm highly concerned and quite wary."

There are three components of the type of therapy Dr. Hamkins and I engage in that I believe helped the most. First, a teamwork mentality exists, so I have felt like I can be more honest with my opinions and I do not feel like demands are being directed at me with an agreement that I will follow the demands exactly. Second, confidentiality here is treated exactly as the definition states, which is seemingly basic, but never achieved with my previous mental health professionals. Lastly, issues faced and ideas discussed are both described so exactly, that the lack of confusion eases the strain of dealing with such complex issues. Dr. Hamkins also does not over simplify possible solutions, which gives me reassurance that the issues I am dealing with are not simple. Being hopeful while maintaining realistic expectations has been found to be a reliable sentiment for our work together.

I do feel like all experiences contain some good and some bad and I feel very privileged to have gained such insight about human suffering and challenges at a young age. It has definitely given me a new perspective on relating to other people and I have great interest in gaining as much knowledge as possible. I have also met incredible people who I never would have, if I didn't go through these challenges.

There are so many aspects of my life now that are positive, that it would be hard to mention them all. Most importantly, I feel the core of my personality is coming back; I do enjoy being the center of attention most times, talking non-stop about everything and anything, and my dry wit humor to name a few aspects. I'm still as stubborn as I was before I became ill, I still hate being in history class or when people use double negatives. I still entertain myself by doing handstands, still believe in angels, and still will not read books if they don't start on page 1. While most of these characteristics are minor, when they are lacking from your life for 8 or 9 years, or just unnoticed, it's a surreal experience when they suddenly reenter your life with a great force. Family and friends are happier because I am happier. I have been able to transfer back to using creativity positively in my life as opposed to obsessing and attempting to break my self-esteem. I do spend a decent amount of time engaging in things that scare me because I know those are the things I'll end up loving the most. I have interests in studying False Memory

Syndrome, feral children, school anxiety, and raising twins, and working with the special needs population and jailed inmates with mental illnesses. I also want to put effort into bridging the gap between psychological and sociological fields. For the first time, I have faith that I can accomplish goals like these.

## Notes

1. Daphne Simeon and Jeffrey Abugel, *Feeling Unreal: Depersonalization Disorder and the Loss of the Self* (London: Oxford University Press, 2008).
2. Jean Frazier, Vice Chair and Director, Division of Child and Adolescent Psychiatry, University of Massachusetts Medical School.
3. Shona Russell, Gaye Stockell, and Peggy Sax, "Replenishing the Spirit of the Work: Rites of Passage" (workshop, Burlington, VT, June 12–14, 2012).

# CONCLUSION

Narrative psychiatry is the North Star that guides me in my work. Whether I am conducting fifteen-minute appointments at a community mental health center, weekly psychotherapy in my private practice, or a college student's first psychiatric consultation, the principles and practices of narrative psychiatry offer me direction and support. In every psychiatric context in which I practice, I seek to enhance my patients' awareness of their strengths and values and assist them in taking steps toward their vision of well-being in the context of a collaborative and compassionate therapeutic relationship.

It's time to bring greater humanity back into the day-to-day practice of psychiatry. Just as primary care practitioners are seeking to attend more fully to their patients' stories and lives, so, too, can we in psychiatry, especially in contexts such as med checks and hospital rounds. Narrative psychiatry offers the person-centered, recovery-oriented care[1] and "positive psychiatry"[2] that the leaders in our field are calling for.

What narrative psychiatry needs to move forward is to train more narrative practitioners and to conduct more research to establish a stronger empirical foundation. Case-based, qualitative evidence of the efficacy of narrative approaches to mental health treatment is rich, such as that presented in this book and in two decades of articles and books published by White, Epston, Madsen, Freedman, Combs, Russell, Gaddis, Kronbichter, Maisel, Ncube, Speedy,[3] and many others. Quantitative studies that have been completed to date, such as Lynette Vromans and Robert Schweitzer's study of narrative treatment of major depression, and Mim Weber, Kierrynn Davis, and Lisa McPhie's study of narrative treat-ment of eating disorders, while supporting efficacy, are limited by small sample sizes.[4]

Exciting research studies are currently underway. John Stillman has developed a narrative trauma treatment manual[5] expressly for the purpose of defining core narrative therapy principles and practices so that their efficacy can be researched. He and Christopher Erbe have completed a pilot study demonstrating the reliability of scales used by observers rating whether therapy sessions were consistent with the practices described by the manual; that is, whether the treatment was actually narrative.[6] With this foundation in place, they have begun studies at the Minneapolis Veterans Affairs Medical Center to determine the effi-cacy of narrative treatment approaches. In a concurrent study in Toronto, Ontario, Laura Béres and Jim Duvall, with Helen Gremillion, Karen Young, and Scot Cooper and consultation support from David Epston, are study-ing process and pivotal moments in narrative therapy and its effects on both patients and therapists.[7] In addition, there is an initiative underway at Providence Behavioral Health Hospital in Holyoke, Massachusetts, led by Beth Prullage,[8] to develop and institute a hospital-wide narrative approach to psychiatric treatment of children and adults, offering a cru-cible in which to further develop and study narrative psychiatry. I look forward to the knowledge we will gain from these endeavors.

The journey of writing this book has been a delight. It has given me the gift of deeply reflecting on my work, discussing it with colleagues, and bringing it out into the world more fully. A particular joy has been sharing with my patients the story of our work together, sending them the chapter in which they are featured, hearing their responses, and, often, bringing their voices forward in writing to add to the book. This writing and reflecting has been a continuation and enrichment of the therapeutic work we had done or are still doing to cultivate stories of strength and meaning.

My hope is that this book will be a springboard for others to take up the ideas and practices of narrative psychiatry and try them out. Let me encourage you to do so.

# Notes

1. Substance Abuse and Mental Health Services Administration, "Recovery Support."
2. American Psychiatric Assocation, "Ingredients of Successful Aging."
3. Michael White, *Narrative Practice: Continuing the Conversations* (New York: W. W. Norton, 2011); White, "Re-engaging with History"; White, *Maps*; White, "Addressing Personal Failure"; White, "Working with People"; White, "Saying Hullo Again"; White, "Pseudo-encopresis"; White and Epston, *Narrative Means*; Madsen, *Collaborative Approaches*; Freedman and Combs, *Narrative Therapy*; Shona Russell, "Deconstructing Perfectionism: Narrative Conversations with Those Suffering from Eating Issues," *International Journal of Narrative Therapy and Community Work* 3 (2007): 21–29; Gaddis, "Repositioning Traditional Research"; Kronbichter, "Narrative Therapy"; Maisel, Epston, and Borden, *Biting the Hand*; Ncube, "Tree of Life"; Speedy, "More Peopled Life."
4. Lynette Vromans and Robert Schweitzer, "Narrative Therapy for Adults with a Major Depressive Disorder: Improved Symptom and Interpersonal Outcomes," *Psychotherapy Research* 21 (2010): 4–15; Mim Weber, Kierrynn Davis, and Lisa McPhie, "Narrative Therapy, Eating Disorders and Groups: Enhancing Outcomes in Rural NSW," *Australian Social Work* 59 no. 4 (2006): 391–405.
5. Stillman, *Trauma Manual*.
6. David Epston, John R. Stillman, and Christopher Erbes, "The Corner: An Innovation in Research in Minnesota; Speaking Two Languages: A Conversation between Narrative Therapy and Scientific Practices," Journal of Systemic Therapies 31 (2012): 74–88.
7. Dulwich Centre, "Research, Evidence and Narrative Practice," accessed January 11, 2013. http://www.dulwichcentre.com.au/narrative-therapy-research.html
8. Beth Prullage, doctoral candidate, Simmons College, Boston, Massachusetts.

# REFERENCES

American Psychiatric Association. *Diagnostic and Statistical Manual of Mental Disorders.* 4th ed., Text Revision. Washington DC: American Psychiatric Association, 2000.

American Psychiatric Association. "Ingredients of Successful Aging Exist Now, Says APA President-Elect." *Psychiatric News Update* 19 (2012). http://www.psychnews.org/update/report1_AM2.html

Anderson, Tom. "The Reflecting Team: Dialogue and Meta-Dialogue in Clinical Work." *Family Process*, 26 (1987): 415–28.

Besa, David. "Evaluating Narrative Family Therapy using Single-System Research Designs." *Research on Social Work Practice*, 4 (1994): 309–25.

Birmingham, Laird, Jenny Su, Julia A. Hlynsky, Eliot M. Goldner, and Min Gao. "The Mortality Rate from Anorexia Nervosa." *International Journal of Eating Disorders* 38 (2005): 143–6. doi:10.1002/eat.20164.

Bruner, Jerome. *Acts of Meaning.* Cambridge, MA: Harvard University Press, 1990.

Bruner, Jerome. *Actual Minds, Possible Worlds.* Cambridge, MA: Harvard University Press, 1987.

Carlat, Daniel. *Unhinged: The Trouble with Psychiatry—A Doctor's Revelations About a Profession in Crisis.* New York: Simon & Schuster, 2010.

Charon, Rita. *Narrative Medicine: Honoring Stories of Illness.* New York: Oxford University Press, 2006.

Crocket, Kathie, Wendy Drewery, Wally McKenzie, Lorraine Smith, and John Winslade. "Working for Ethical Research in Practice." *International Journal of Narrative Therapy and Community Work* 3 (2004): 61–66.

Dreyfuss, Claudia, ed.. *Seizing Our Bodies: The Politics of Women's Health.* New York: Vintage Books, 1977.

Dulwich Centre. "Companions on a Journey: An Exploration of an Alternative Community Mental Health Project." *Dulwich Centre Newsletter* 1 (1997): 2–36.

Dulwich Centre. "Research, Evidence and Narrative Practice." Accessed January 11, 2013. http://www.dulwichcentre.com.au/narrative-therapy-research.html

Dulwich Centre Publications. "Narrative Therapy and Research." *International Journal of Narrative Therapy and Community Work* 2 (2004), 29–36.

Epston, David, John R. Stillman, and Christopher Erbes. "The Corner: An Innovation in Research in Minnesota; Speaking Two Languages: A Conversation between Narrative Therapy and Scientific Practices." *Journal of Systemic Therapies* 31 (2012): 74–88.

Foucault, Michel. *Discipline and Punish: The Birth of the Prison*. Translated by Alan Sheridan. New York: Random House, 1979. First published in French as *Surveiller et Punir: Naissance de la prison*. Paris: Editions Gallimard, 1975.

Foucault, Michel. *The History of Madness*. Edited by Jean Khalfa, translated by Jonathan Murphy. Abingdon, UK: Routledge, 2006. First published in French as *Folie et déraison: Histoire de la folie à l'âge classique*. Paris: Librarie Plon, 1961.

Foucault, Michel. *The History of Sexuality, Volume I: An Introduction*. Translated by Robert Hurley. New York: Random House, 1978. First published in French as *La volenté de savoir*. Paris: Editions Gallimard, 1976.

Foucault, Michel. *Madness and Civilization: A History of Insanity in the Age of Reason*. New York: Random House, 1965.

Freedman, Jill, and Gene Combs. *Narrative Therapy: The Social Construction of Preferred Realities*. New York: W.W. Norton, 1996.

Gaddis, Stephen. "Repositioning Traditional Research: Centering Clients' Accounts in the Construction of Professional Therapy Knowledges." *International Journal of Narrative Therapy and Community Work* 2 (2004), 37–48.

Goren-Watts, Rachael "Eating Disorder Metaphors: A Qualitative Meta-synthesis of Women's Experiences." PhD diss., Antioch University New England, Keene, NH, 2011.

Greely, Henry, Barbara Sahakian, John Harris, Ronald C. Kessler, and Michael Gazzaniga. "Toward Responsible Use of Cognitive-Enhancing Drugs by the Healthy." *Nature* 456 (December 10, 2008): 702–5.

Hamkins, SuEllen. "Bringing Narrative Practices to Psychopharmacology." *The International Journal of Narrative Therapy and Community Work* 1 (2010): 56–71.

———. "Introducing Narrative Psychiatry: Narrative Approaches to Initial Psychiatric Consultations." *The International Journal of Narrative Therapy and Community Work* 1 (2005): 5–17.

Hare-Muston, Rachel. "Discourses in the Mirrored Room: A Postmodern Analysis of Therapy." *Family Process*, 33 (1994): 35.

Joffe-Walt, Chana. "Unfit for Work: The Startling Rise of Disability in America." National Public Radio. Accessed April 15, 2013, http://apps.npr.org/unfit-for-work/.

Kirsch, Irving. *The Emperor's New Drugs: Exploding the Antidepressant Myth*. New York: Basic Books, 2010.

Kirsch, Irving, Brett J. Deacon, Tania Huedo-Medina, Alan Scoboria, Thomas Moore, and Blair T. Johnson. "Initial Severity and Antidepressant Benefits: A Meta-analysis of Data Submitted to the Food and Drug Administration." *PLoS Med* 5, no. 2 (2008): e45. doi:10.1371/journal.pmed.0050045.

Kronbichter, Rudi. "Narrative Therapy with Boys Struggling with Anorexia." *International Journal of Narrative Therapy and Community Work* 4 (2004): 55–70.

Lewis, Bradley. *Narrative Psychiatry: How Stories Can Shape Clinical Practice*. Baltimore: Johns Hopkins University Press, 2011.

Linehan, Marcia. *Cognitive-Behavioral Treatment of Borderline Personality Disorder*. New York: Guilford, 1993.

Madsen, William. *Collaborative Therapy with Multi-stressed Families*. 2nd ed. New York: Guilford, 2007.

Maisel, Richard, David Epston, and Alison Borden. *Biting the Hand That Starves You*. New York: W.W. Norton, 2004.

Mehl-Madrona, Lewis. *Healing the Mind through the Power of Story: The Promise of Narrative Psychiatry*. Rochester, VT: Bear, 2010.

Morgan, Robin, ed. *Sisterhood Is Powerful* New York: Random House, 1970.

Myerhoff, Barbara. *Number Our Days* New York: Touchstone Books, 1979.

Ncube, Ncazelo. "The Journey of Healing: Using Narrative Therapy and Map-Making to Respond to Child-Abuse in South Africa." *International Journal of Narrative Therapy and Community Work* 1 (2010): 3–12.

Ncube, Ncazelo. The Tree of Life Project: Using Narrative Ideas in Work with Vulnerable Children in Southern Africa. *International Journal of Narrative Therapy and Community Work* 1 (2006): 3–16.

Rich, Adrienne. *Blood, Bread and Poetry: Selected Prose 1979-1985*. New York: W. W. Norton, 1986.

Ricoeur, Paul. *From Text to Action: Essays in Hermeneutics, II*. Translated by Kathleen Blamey and John B. Thompson. Evanston, IL: Northwestern University Press, 1991. (First published in French as *Du texts a l'action: Eassia d'hermeneutique, II* by Editions due Seuil, 1986.)

Roth, Sallyann, and Richard Chasin. "Entering One Another's Worlds of Meaning and Imagination: Dramatic Enactment and Narrative Couple Therapy," in *Constructive Therapies*, Vol. 1, edited by Michael Hoyt, 189–216. New York: Guilford, 1994.

Roth, Sallyann, and David Epston. "Consulting the Problem about the Problematic Relationship: An Exercise for Experiencing a Relationship with an Externalized Problem," In *Constructive Therapies*, Vol. 2, edited by Michael Hoyt, 148–62. New York: Guilford, 1996.

Russell, Shona. "Deconstructing Perfectionism: Narrative Conversations with Those Suffering from Eating Issues." *International Journal of Narrative Therapy and Community Work* 3 (2007): 21–29.

Russell, Shona, Gaye Stockell, and Peggy Sax. "Replenishing the Spirit of the Work: Rites of Passage." Workshop, Burlington, VT, June 12–14, 2012.

Schechter, Richard. *Essays in Performance Theory*. New York: Ralph Pine, for Drama School Specialists, 1977.

Seikkula, Jaako. "Five-Year Experience of First-Episode Nonaffective Psychosis Treated in Open-Dialogue Approach: Treatment Principles, Follow-Up Outcomes, and Two Case Studies." *Psychotherapy Research* 16 (2006): 214–28.

Siegel, Daniel J. *The Mindful Therapist: A Clinician's Guide to Mindsight and Neural Integration*. New York: W. W. Norton and Company, 2010.

Simeon, Daphne, and Jeffrey Abugel. *Feeling Unreal: Depersonalization Disorder and the Loss of the Self*. London: Oxford University Press, 2008.

Speedy, Jane. "Living a More Peopled Life: Definitional Ceremony As Inquiry into Psychotherapy 'Outcomes.'" *International Journal of Narrative Therapy and Community Work* 3 (2004): 43–53.

Stillman, John. *Narrative Therapy Trauma Manual: A Principle-Based Approach*. St. Louis Park, MN: Casperson, 2012.

Substance Abuse and Mental Health Services Administration. "Recovery Support." Accessed January 11, 2013. .

Substance Abuse and Mental Health Services Administration. "SAMHSA's Working Definition of Recovery from Mental Disorders and Substance Use Disorders." *SAMHSA Blog*. December 22, 2011. http://blog.samhsa.gov/2011/12/22/samhsa%E2%80%99s-definition-and-guiding-principles-of-recovery-%E2%80%93-answering-the-call-for-feedback/.

Substance Abuse and Mental Health Services Administration. "Welcome to the National Center for Trauma-Informed Care." Accessed January 11, 2013. http://www.samhsa.gov/nctic/default.asp.

Tootell, Andrew. "Decentring Research Practice." *International Journal of Narrative Therapy and Community Work* 3 (2004): 54–55.

Vromans, Lynette, and Robert Schweitzer. "Narrative Therapy for Adults with a Major Depressive Disorder: Improved Symptom and Interpersonal Outcomes." *Psychotherapy Research* 21 (2010): 4–15. doi:10.1080/10503301003591792.

Walker, Alice. *In Search of Our Mothers' Gardens.* New York: Harcourt Brace Jovanovich, 1984.

Watters, Ethan. *Crazy Like Us: The Globalization of the American Psyche.* New York: Free Press, 2010.

Weber, Mim, Kierrynn Davis, and Lisa McPhie. "Narrative Therapy, Eating Disorders and Groups: Enhancing Outcomes in Rural NSW." *Australian Social Work* 59 no. 4 (2006): 391–405. .

Whitaker, Robert. *Anatomy of an Epidemic: Magic Bullets, Psychiatric Drugs, and the Astonishing Rise of Mental Illness in America.* New York: Crown, 2010.

White, Michael. "Addressing Personal Failure." *The International Journal of Narrative Therapy and Community Work* 3 (2002), 33–76.

White, Michael. *Maps of Narrative Practice.* New York: W.W. Norton, 2007.

White, Michael. *Narrative Practice: Continuing the Conversations.* New York: W. W. Norton, 2011.

White, Michael. "Pseudo-encopresis: From Avalanche to Victory, from Vicious to Virtuous Cycles." *Family Systems Medicine* 2 (1984): 150–60.

White, Michael. "Re-authoring Conversations." Workshop presented at the Family Institute of New Jersey, March 15, 1997.

White, Michael. *Re-authoring Lives: Interviews and Essays.* Adelaide, Australia: Dulwich Centre Publications, 1995.

White, Michael. "Re-engaging with History: The Absent but Implicit." In *Reflections on narrative practice: Essays and interviews*, edited by Michael White, 35–58. Adelaide, Australia: Dulwich Centre Publications, 2000.

White, Michael. "Saying Hullo Again: The Incorporation of the Lost Relationship in the Resolution of Grief." *Dulwich Centre Newsletter* Spring (1988), 7–11.

White, Michael. *Selected Papers.* Adelaide, Australia: Dulwich Centre Publications, 1989.

White, Michael. "Working with People Who Are Suffering the Consequences of Multiple Trauma: A Narrative Perspective." *The International Journal of Narrative Therapy and Community Work* 1 (2004), 45–76.

White, Michael, and David Epston. *Narrative Means to Therapeutic Ends.* New York: W.W. Norton, 1990.

White, Michael, and Alice Morgan. *Narrative Therapy with Children and Their Families.* Adelaide, Australia: Dulwich Centre Publications, 2006.

Woolf, Virginia. *A Room of One's Own.* New York and London: Harcourt Brace Jovanovich, 1929.

# INDEX

Made in the USA
Middletown, DE
15 June 2017